# INTERMITTENT FASTING

Fasting and eating for health. Control your weight with healthy food, reset your metabolism thanks to fasting. Burn fat and enjoy your new diet

KAITLYN TERRELL

# Contents

# What is fasting?

Fasting – Staying without food for a certain period. There are different fasting methods and types. In some, you have to avoid food and water for several hours, whereas some fasting methods allow liquids. Different fasting methods have various benefits, but the most common thing about all the fasting methods "it is good for physical and mental health" typically fasting is done for religious purposes. Many religions, including Christianity and Islam, refrain people from eating anything from dusk to dawn. People from different faiths believe that fasting filters out all the toxic elements from your body and helps in keeping body and mind fresh. Well, this has also been proven with the help of certain studies, that fasting burns fats and reduces the risks of diseases, especially heart diseases.

People fasts for different reasons, it might be a type of dieting for some, and others do it because it is part of their spiritual journey. People usually confuse fasting with starving. Fasting doesn't mean to starve to death and to say goodbye to all your favorite foods. But it demands you to avoid food for certain hours and then eat healthy in the non-fasting hours. During non-fasting hours, you can eat whatever you like the most as long as you are eating healthy and nutritious food.

Recent studies and researches have shown that fasting is one of the best ways to reduce stress and helps people fighting with mental toughness. It is because it boosts up brain activity and makes it even sharp and smart. Let's talk about fasting as a part of religion first.

## Fasting in Bible

Christianity, the first largest religion of the world that has millions of people as followers are bound to fast according to their holy book bible. Fasting is the part of their faith, and Christians believe that they are answerable to God about fasting.

The Bible likewise gives guidelines about the mentality and approach we ought to have in fasting. Jesus cautioned about two-faced fasting, attempting to flaunt or cause others to feel sorry for us (Matthew

6:16-17). Rather we ought not "appear to men too quickly, yet to your Father who is in the mystery place" (section 18).

The method of fasting is different in Christianity. You can drink water and even juices while fasting but avoiding food cooked on the fire for several hours.

Everything that is the part of religion and that is assigned to humans by God, must have a lot of advantages. Not only religion but fasting is also an important factor in health science, and according to health experts, fasting has different kinds.

## Fasting in Islam:

Islam is the second-largest religion of the world, with millions of followers found at every corner across the globe. People following Islam are generally known as "Muslims," and fasting is the one major part of their lives. Muslims believe that fasting is very important to complete their spiritual journey, and it strengthens their relationship with God. But their religion has confined fasting to only one month in a year. The fasting month is known as "Ramzan," and it consists of either 30 or 29 days. Muslims are bound to keep themselves away from any kind of food and drink that gives energy to the body. Their fast is mostly 12-14 hours long, and they believe it filters out all the non-toxic items from their mind and body. Research has shown, individuals who fast during the month of Ramzan are more healthy and have less risk of physical and mental diseases.

No matter what kind of fast you are practice, but in the end, the main purpose of fasting is "Cleansing and Detoxifying."

## Cleansing and Detoxifying

A wide range of fasting gives a similarly large number of advantages. You don't have to do a fast with "purify" or "detox" in it, to free your body of undesirable poisons or toxic elements. Nor do you have to do a "profound" fast to profit yourself spiritually. No matter what, but a wide range of fasting will lead you on the way to better and higher spots.

Though the main purpose of every fast is to detox your body. So it is now important to select the kind and type of fasting that suits best to your body and its requirements. Fasting without research or preparations might lead you towards serious health hazards. That's why selecting the right kind of fasting, and discussing it with your health expert is very important. Many people have to face severe migraines and nausea even in the starting hours of fasting; it is because they lack the basic preparations and practice fast out of nowhere. I would suggest you start with an easier kind of fasting. It will prepare your body for further fasting and also starts the detox process.

Also, take a lot of low sugary juices and water during fasting hours. It speeds up the cleansing process and detoxes your body fastly. Drinking a lot of fluid during fasting hours is also helpful in cleaning the stomach and kidneys.

Let's talk about fasting and its methods, according to health experts all across the globe. Read them out and select the one that suits best to your body requirements.

# Kinds of fasting

Fasting is not only ignoring food and energetic items for a certain period. Glancing back at our base beginnings, fasting was a piece of regular daily existence. During this time, it was a test to source our nourishments, and along these lines, it was typical to avoid food for a certain timeframe. Quick forward to the 21st century and sourcing nourishment is not a big issue at all. Now we can do whatever we want and whenever we want by just clicking a button on our phone screens.

With this new period in nourishment sourcing, our storerooms and refrigerators are as full as could be. However, simultaneously, fasting has picked up prominence and is now retouched as a 'speedy' hack to achieve a healthy body and healthy mind.

There are different kinds of fasting. That is further divided into several fasting methods. Different individuals have different body potentials. All kinds of fasting methods are not suitable for everyone. That's why fasting is divided into three main kinds. You can select the best one that suits your body or take the help of your doctor or health expert.

The following are three main kinds of fasting. Let's explore them together.

- *Macro-nutrient restriction fasting*
- *Calorie restriction fasting*
- *Seasonal fasting*

Let's talk about Micronutrient fasting first.

# Macro-nutrient restriction fasting

This sort of fast includes confining a certain macronutrient (The three macronutrients are proteins, starches, and fats). Commonly these fasts are protein de-loads. These kinds of fasts work best for competitors, sportspersons, or athletes who have a higher protein necessity and are reliably focusing on their guts. In this kind of fasting, individuals will only intake top-notch fats, carbohydrates, and completely cooked vegetables for 2-3 days in a month. The decrease in protein utilization will offer the gut a reprieve and permit it to mend. Remember that it is as yet imperative to ensure that their activity is insignificant during this timeframe. It is recommended to avoid all the extra efforts during this kind of fasting because your body is already running low at some nutrition.

# Calorie restriction fasting

The essential kind of fasting is a calorie limitation of fasting. This is the thing that a great many people consider when they hear the expression "fasting." It is essentially abandoning nourishment for a specific timeframe. These sorts of fasts are commonly done between 18-48 hours. To benefit from this kind of fasting, it is important to ensure whoever is fasting has devoured sufficient calories for a certain period. At that point, pick a day, have supper early, and fast for the assigned time. During the fast, just expend water and keep activity levels low to help the fasted state. It is suggested to avoid hectic activities like sports, a lot of exercise, and other exhausting activities in the beginning time. Because the body has already restricted calories, so it may affect your health in negative manners.

This type of fasting is also known as "intermittent fasting" or " irregular fasting." it is further divided into different forms. (we will discuss it later)

# Seasonal fasting

The third sort of fasting is not a typical fast by any means; it's occasional eating. For this sort of fast, we should glance back at basic occasions and inspect what our nourishment supply would have resembled during various seasons like winters, summers, autumn, and spring. In the winter, fattier meats and tubers were expended, and summer was held for products of the soil like fresh fruits and vegetables and some amount of meats. To genuinely eat occasionally, just eat what might normally be accessible during that season. Most human advancements at northern scopes wouldn't approach ready bananas in January. Regular eating follows the idea of customized nourishment, realizing what works best for you.

God hasn't created anything that is not beneficial for human beings. All seasonal foods are best for human physical and mental health. So if you are a diet conscious person but fasting is not your cup of tea, then eating seasonal foods is the best choice for you.

Some other famous kinds of fasting are as follows:

## Juices and Fruits Fasts:

Juices and fruits fasting is useful for beginners. This kind of fasting allows the intake of a certain amount of fresh juices. It could be vegetable juices or fresh fruit juices or a combination of both. During the fasting hours, it is recommended to take a lot of juices and clean water. It gives you nutrition and vitamins and, at the same time, helps the body in cleansing and detoxifying. Fresh juices are good for mental and physical health. They are not heavy on the stomach but still gives you the energy to perform your daily chores. The best thing is to use seasonal fruits and vegetables.

The quickest way of making fresh juice is.

- Take some fresh fruits and vegetables and peel them off carefully.
- Now cut the small pieces and add them to the grinder.
- Add a glass of water, with a pinch of salt and sugar, to maintain the body's sugar and salt level.
- Add some ice to make it rich and tasty.

If you don't like juices much, no worries, you can also eat a lot of raw fruits and vegetables.

## Water fasting

Of all the different kinds of fasting, water fasting is the oldest form of fasting. As the name suggests, this kind of fasting is about drinking clean water for a certain period. It could be several hours before breakfast or sometimes in the evening, depending upon your convenience and ease. Water fasting is best for cleaning your kidneys and stomach. It prevents your body from dehydration and keeps you active throughout the day. In my opinion, this is one of the easiest yet effective ways of fasting.

## Diagnostic fasts:

This is a different kind of fast that is only performed by some specific individuals. Like people who are undergoing some kind of surgery or any medical test. During this kind of fast, intake of food or any kind of liquid is completely banned until a certain function is performed. For instance, before the lipid profile test, it is important to fast for at least 10-12 hours. In some cases, even water is not allowed during fasting hours.

## Fast mimicking

It is an altered kind of fasting. Some probably won't think of it as fasting by any means, yet to a greater extent, it is somewhat related to a calorie limited fasting. Fast mimicking includes eating modest quantities over some period, which is regularly five days. The eating regimen is generally high in fats and low in protein and sugars.

It was intended to be more feasible than specific types of fasting. However, a few people could battle with the continuous calorie confined to nature. Somebody types work perfectly with only one fasting window instead of five days back to back long periods of fasting

The general goal of this kind of fasting is to get the advantages from customary sorts of fasting, yet without totally cutting yourself off nourishment. Studies on this one are restricted. However, early research recommends some similar advantages to the typical type of fasting.

# Intermittent Fasting

With the passing days, we can see a modification in almost everything. The same is the case with fasting as well. Intermittent fasting is also known as "irregular fasting," and it is one of the most common forms of fasting nowadays. Though it has many different methods depending upon fasting hours and intake of calories, here I am going to discuss the 7 best ways of intermittent fasting.

## o *12 hours of fasting*

This is a simple fasting technique, in which you are required to fast for 12 hours in a day. You can select any consecutive 12 hours as a fasting window and the rest of the hours as an eating window. According to health experts, fasting for 10-12 hours helps to burn stored body fats, and in return, they turn them into energy. This energy is released in the body as ketones, and it serves as the basic element that helps in weight loss.

This fasting routine is good for beginners. That is because the fasting hours are equal to the eating window. Also, 8-10 fasting hours easily go during sleep. It means you are only fasting for 4-6 hours. That is a perfect window for the beginners. Twelve hours of fasting also is useful in restricting calorie intake. It has a lot of positive health impacts, and all of the above, it helps in weight reduction, control diseases; it is good for mental health and improves metabolism.

## o *16 hours of fasting*

This method is very famous and commonly known as the 16:8 method. It means you have to fast for 16 hours with 8 hours eating window. Once you have started with 12 hours of fasting, it is easy for you to move forward towards the 16:8 method as your body is already used to fasting. For women, it is recommended to take 500 calories during fasting hours, whereas men are supposed to take around 600 calories. You can have light sugary juices and some raw fruits and vegetables to maintain your energy during fasting hours.

16:8 methods are very helpful for people suffering from obesity. Researches and studies have shown that this method is quite useful in weight reduction and has a lot of other positive health impacts as well.

## o *2 days fasting:*

This diet plan is about eating healthy 5 days a week and fasting for the rest of 2 days. By fasting, here means to restrict calories to 500-600 per day only. This diet is also popular with the name "the Fast Diet," and it was first introduced by a British man "Michael Mosley." It is reported that the 5:2 diet plan is one of the most effective ways of reducing weight and helps to get a better lifestyle. The 5:2 diet plan doesn't restrict you from the number of calories you intake. Or it is not about what foods you are eating.

This diet plan also allows you to take 500-600 calories to avoid body collapse and other harmful effects of intermittent fasting. Though there isn't very much research on the 5:2 method of fasting, some research has shown that it is quite helpful in weight reduction. A study conducted on 102 obese people practicing the 5:2 method for a few weeks has shown positive results of weight reduction.

o ***Alternate Day Fasting:***

Alternate day fasting, as the name suggests, is the fasting method that requires a 24-hours fast every alternate day. This method is not recommended for beginners, as it is not an easy one. If you want to lose weight and improve body metabolism, then alternate day fasting is a good choice. On fasting day, you are only allowed to intake 500-600 calories along with some low-fat juices, coffee, and a lot of water.

Studies have shown that alternate-day fasting is very useful for heart health and weight reduction. Research conducted on 32 overweight people showed that practicing alternate-day fasting results in a loss of 5.2 kgs.

## o *A 24 hour fast:*

Fasting completely for a day or two is known as the eat stop eat method of fasting. In this method, you are required to fast for 24 hours with little intake of juices and 25% of total calories. It could be lunch-lunch, dinner-dinner, breakfast-breakfast kind of fasting. You can select any 24 hours that are convenient for you. This method of fasting is not recommended for beginners, though. As it is a tough and hectic method and needs a lot of patience and tolerance. Eat stop eat method of fasting does wonder when we talk about weight reduction and better health.

## o *The warrior method*

As the name suggests, this diet plan has got some inspiration from the ancient warriors. The warriors back then used to eat a little amount of food during the day time and eat good healthy foods at night to fulfill the body's nutritional requirements and to stay healthy and active. This fasting method requires you to eat some raw fruit and vegetables during the day time and eat one good healthy processed meal at night. This method is an easy way for beginners who are trying to lose weight but in an easy manner.

This diet plan mainly focuses on fasting for 20 hours a day, by fasting here means you can have small meals during the day time, like eating raw fruits, or dairy products like milk and boiled eggs and after they complete 24 hours eat as much as you want but eat healthy meals consist up of all the proteins and vitamins.

## o *Meal Skipping*

This is the easiest and convenient approach for beginners. It suggests skipping meals whenever it is easy for you. You have to decide which meal to skip, depending upon your food and hunger requirements. In addition to that, it is very important to eat healthy food in other meals as well.

Meal skipping method is also useful in weight loss and improves body and mind health.

Fasting isn't for everybody, and before you start confining your eating, there are a few requirements to remember. If you are not following the rules and regulations related to fasting, tell me what is the point of fasting then? So let's talk about the prerequisite of fasting.

# Prerequisite of fasting:

To get all benefits out of fasting, it is important to recall the following prequels of fasting in your mind again and again.

**Self-discipline:** it is important to discipline your life once you have started fasting. By discipline, I mean to get everything on point, like sleeping on time, waking up early in the morning. Set your suppers timings properly. Get good sleep, healthy food, and a little workout. Once you have discipline in your life, it would be easier for you to get the desired results.

**Self-control:** Self-control means to avoid junk food or unhealthy food and to control your habits of eating junk. Unhealthy eating kills the purpose of fasting, and you may end up having no benefits out of it.

**Self-motivation:** motivation is another important prerequisite of fasting. Motive yourself to stick to the fasting routine. There is no point in fasting if you are doing it without any motivation. Watch inspirational videos on YouTube or ask your friends to boost your confidence in you. A healthy conversation between your loved ones might help you in getting the desired motivation.

# Tips for choosing the right fasting method for you

As I have mentioned earlier, it is important to choose the right method of fasting for yourself. Here are some tips that would be helpful for you to select the right kind of fasting.

The most important thing is to ask yourself

- Either you are experienced? Or are you trying it for the first time?

- Your body habits and medical status. People with medical history are not recommended to start fasting without concerning their health experts.

- What kind of fast do you want? A long term or a short term?

- What is the objective of fasting? And what are you trying to achieve?

- Your lifestyle? What are your responsibilities and commitments? Is it possible for you to fast successfully or not?

Once you have the answer to all these questions, it will become easier for you to select the right kind of fasting for yourself.

# How to fast safely?

Fasting could be quite dangerous if not done properly. In addition to that, always remember that fasting is not for everyone. If you have any medical history, you need to concern the doctor before starting practicing it.

Following people should avoid fasting without the doctor's advice.

- People with a medical history including heart disease or type 2 diabetes
- Women who are trying to conceive
- Women who are pregnant
- Breastfeeding women
- Underweight individuals.
- People suffering from an eating disorder
- People who have problems with blood sugar regulation
- individuals with low blood pressure
- Those who are taking prescription medications

- Woman with a history of amenorrhea

- Older adults

- Adolescents

- People suffering from depression or anxiety.

- People with a weak immune system.

- Women who are on their periods. As periods make the body dull and weaker, that makes it difficult to sustain the fast.

If you are healthy and do not belong to the category of people mentioned above, then you are okay to start fasting. But here are some tips that can make your fasting safe and beneficial.

## Start with short fasting periods

As I have mentioned a lot of ways of fasting, and you are free to select the one. I would suggest you select the one with shorter fasting periods. It could be 4-5 hours. Give your body some time to get settled with your new fasting routine. Jumping straight towards

12-24 hours fast might lead you towards body collapse, dehydration, or other health hazards. That's why the most important thing to keep in your mind is, keep the duration short. Begin with the shorter period and then extend it step by step.

## Take a few calories during fasting hours

In the beginning, it is allowed to take 25% of calories during fasting hours. It makes 500-600 calories. The best way to take these calories is in the form of low sugary juices. Fresh juices are the best ways to keep you hydrated and also gives you enough energy to complete your fast successfully.

Cutting down the entire food intake at once might affect your body or brain. Some people feel migraine and nausea during the hours of fasting. That's because their body is not used to it. Once you got used to your fasting routine, cut down the extra calories. At that moment, it would not bother you that much.

Precisely we can say that eating a small amount on fast days rather than cutting out all food helps reduce your risk of side effects. And you don't feel hungry all the time.

## Meditate

Meditation is one useful activity that helps divert your mind. It is very important to find out ways that can kill boredom and distract your mind. Otherwise, you might end up thinking about "food" all day. Meditation is also helpful in soothing your mind and brain. If you are feeling Castaic or fasting seems hectic to you. Don't worry. Sit down in the back garden of your house. Feel the peace and inhale a good amount of air. Now count from 1-10 and exhale the air. This activity is good for distracting your mind and helps you to sustain your fast in a better way.

You don't need hours and hours for meditation; just 10 minutes meditation is enough for one day.

## Stay Hydrated:

As 20-30% of water comes from food while fasting, your body is already missing this percentage of water. Health experts suggest drinking coffee and some other healthy low-fat juices during fasting to avoid the risk of dehydration. Also, it helps you to sustain fasting more effectively. Fasting for a long period might result in dehydration, headaches, dry lips, and throats, and fatigue. So, the best way to avoid all these things is to drink a lot of water and keep yourself hydrated. According to some health experts, it is important to drink 2-3 liters of water every day (14 glasses of water); otherwise, there might be a risk of body collapse.

Drinking a lot of water during fasting hours also helps in triggering the cleaning process of the body. So stay hydrated, fresh and active during the fasting hours, to get great benefit out of fasting.

## Walk or Mild Exercise:

Some people think that they can manage their exercise schedules even during fasting hours. Though They Might be right, doctors and health experts suggest rescheduling your exercise hours during fasting time. Intense or heavy workouts are dangerous for health, and it can cause body collapse at once. As your body is running low on nutrition and fluids. It Doesn't Have the same level of energy. In some cases, intense exercise also results in severe dehydration, muscle pull, and migraine. That's why it is important to reduce your workout hours and keep it mild and safe.

Many experts, on the other hand, suggest an evening or morning walk. A 15-20 minutes walk is enough to keep you fresh and active even during fasting hours. Also, walking with friends could be a fun activity to avoid "food thoughts" now and then.

## Breakfast if feeling unwell:

Though fasting is good for health, it doesn't mean every person can do every kind of fasting. Before fasting, it is important to study and observe your body or to consult some health experts or doctors. No matter if you are 20 years old or you are 85 years, it is important to observe your body and its capabilities. Fasting is good for health; all of us already know that, but breaking a fast isn't any kind. In case you are feeling nauseated, or having a severe headache or any other illness, it is okay to break the fast at every moment and take some healthy food as soon as possible. Nothing is more important than your life.

Sometimes staying hungry for longer periods makes you nauseated or weak. In this situation, it is okay to break a fast by eating something healthy and nutritious.

Seek medical help if important or consider some food supplements too.

In addition to that, only start fasting once you feel healthy and fresh. Sometimes we woke up lazy and tired in the morning. If it's the case with you, then that is not a fasting day at all.

## Take a healthy Diet:

Healthy meals mean foods that are enriched with lots of nutrition, fibers, good fats, calcium, and minerals. That keeps your body active and healthy. All these foods are human-friendly and have a lot of health benefits if taken in a proper proportion. You can ensure you're eating good meals and stay sound by picking entire nourishments like meat, fish, eggs, vegetables, foods grown from the ground when you eat. Whole food regimens dependent on entire nourishments are connected to a wide scope of medical advantages, including a diminished danger of malignancy, coronary illness, and other ceaseless diseases. Try to eat food enriched in proteins. Proteins give your body energy to stay active even during fasting hours, and you are then capable of performing daily responsibilities in a better way. In addition to that, some studies suggest that consuming around 30% of a meal's calories from protein can help in reducing your appetite as well. So the intake of a good amount of protein can help in reducing the side effects of fasting as well.

Precisely, the main purpose of fasting is to improve your health and to stay active. Even though fasting includes going without nourishment, it's as yet essential to keep up a whole food on days when you are not fasting.

## Take multivitamins

Taking a multivitamin is constantly a smart thought, in that it gives you an increase in supplements you may not be getting enough of through eating alone. Although doctors suggest taking multivitamins even in daily routine, it becomes much more necessary during fasting routine. For a powerful mix that will normally bolster your vitality levels, go for Vitacost Synergy Multivitamin. Providing 22 fundamental nutrients and minerals, including nutrient D, folate, and zinc, this hotshot item likewise contains green group CoQ10 and other health benefits, including strong cell reinforcements.

## Avoid junk and heavy feasts:

Many people are mistaken that they can eat whatever they want during a non-fasting window. That is not true in any case. It is very important to eat healthy food enriched with proteins, fibers, calcium, and fats and to avoid all the junk and oily feasts. Many

Individuals, after fasting for long hours, usually break their fast with a heavy feast, which is not good for their health at all. In addition to that, unhealthy eating also kills the basic purpose of fasting. Eating heavy and unhealthy food after fasting may lead you towards dizziness, and you might feel tired. It will make your body inactive. And it would not help you in the weight loss process as well.

Fasting has dozens of health benefits if it is done in the right way. The above tips are to avoid the side effects of fasting. They Might be helpful for you to follow the right rules and regulations of fasting. Remember that nothing is more important than your safety. So keep yourself safe even during fasting hours.

Food Guide: What to eat and what to avoid during fasting

The main purpose of fasting is to be "healthy" and to lose some "extra pounds." There is no point in staying hungry for hours and hours if you are not able to control your diet and maintain your health. The most important thing is to make it clear in your mind what to eat and what not to eat once you have selected any particular type of fasting for yourself. Here is a brief guide of eating healthy and reducing extra weight to get the best benefits out of fasting.

*Your daily diet should contain the following nutrition:*

## ✓ Proteins:

Your body requirement of protein may vary depending upon your fitness goals. But according to health experts, the recommended dietary allowance of protein is 0.8 grams of your total weight. Intake of a suitable amount of protein during your daily routine helps in the weight reduction process, as it fulfills the body's energy demands, and at the same time, it helps in improving metabolism. Especially for the individuals who are practicing exercise and gym along with fasting should try to maintain body protein level, because it is good for muscular mass. In addition to that, proteins cause weight reduction without affecting muscular mass. According to recent research conducted on muscular mass, it has been proved that having more muscle mass on legs helps in the reduction of belly fats, especially in men.

So here, I have selected the list of foods that you should have while practicing a fasting routine. These foods are protein enriched and also help in the weight reduction process during fasting.

- Poultry and fish
- Eggs
- Seafood
- Dairy products including milk, yogurt, and cheese
- Seeds and nuts
- Beans and legumes
- Soy
- A lot of Whole grains

## ✓ Fats:

As all of us know, excess fats in the body are harmful to health. It leads to many dangerous diseases like heart attack and high levels of cholesterol. But according to some health experts, a human body should at least take 20-30% of fats in daily routine. This ratio might vary depending upon your fitness routine and body weight. On the other hand, it is recommended to take only 10% of saturated fats. There are two kinds of fats, good fats, and bad fats. Bad fats are those which are stored in the human body and result in diseases, including weight gain. Meanwhile, good fats are important to give the body some energy and keep it active and fresh. Saturated fats can build the danger of coronary illness. Nonetheless, many health experts have differences of opinion on this matter. It's insightful to eat them with some restraint. Red meat, milk, coconut oil, and bakery items contain high measures of bad or saturated fats.

Solid fats incorporate monounsaturated and polyunsaturated fats. These fats can lessen the danger of coronary illness, lower circulatory strain, and diminish the blood levels of fats.

- Olive oil
- peanut oil
- canola oil
- safflower oil
- sunflower oil
- and soybean oils

The above all are rich sources of good fats.
Following fats, enriched foods are recommended to eat.

- Avocados
- Nuts
- Cheese

- Whole eggs

- Dark chocolate

- Fatty fish

- Chia seeds

- Extra virgin olive oil

- Full-fat yogurt

## ✓ Carbs

Carbohydrates are an important part of the human body. Carbs help to keep the body active and healthy and fight against many diseases. According to health experts, our body needs 45-65% carbs of total calorie intake. Carbs are a significant source of energy for the human body. The other two are protein and fat. Carbs come in different structures. The most prominent of them are sugar, fiber, and starch.

Carbs frequently get negative criticism for causing weight gain. But not all carbs are made equivalent, and they are not innately swelling. Regardless of whether you will put on weight relies upon the sort and amount of the carbs you eat. Make a point to pick nourishments that are high in fiber and starch; however, low in sugar. A recent report recommends that eating 30 grams of fiber every day can cause weight reduction, improve glucose levels, and lower circulatory strain.

Getting 30 grams of fiber from your eating regimen isn't a tough thing. You can get them by eating

- A basic egg sandwich
- Mediterranean grain with chickpeas
- apple with nutty spread
- chicken and dark peas.

The following foods are enriched with carbs that you must intake while practicing a fasting routine.

- Apples
- Berries
- Kidney beans
- Pears

- Avocado

- Carrots

- Broccoli

- Brussels sprouts

- Almonds

- Chia seeds

- Chickpeas

- Sweet potatoes

- Beetroots

- Quinoa

- Oats

- Brown rice

- Bananas

- Mangoes

- Apples

## ✓ Hydration:

Water is very important. In addition to water, some other fluids are recommended to take to keep your body hydrated and avoid the side effects of fasting on your body. If you are taking all the healthy meals in a day but ignoring the good intake of water, I tell you it's not good for your health at all. The human body has 97% water, and it is very important to keep yourself hydrated. According to health experts, the total body requirement of water is

- About 15.5 cups (3.7 liters) for men.
- About 11.5 cups (2.7 liters) for women.

Dehydration is very dangerous for the human body. Severe dehydration, if not handled properly, sometimes results in death as well. Other dangers of dehydration include.

- Diarrhea
- Nausea.
- Severe headache, migraine,
- Body pain,
- Dizziness and tiredness.
- Dullness and lack of energy to do anything.
- Slows down your brain.

In case you are already suffering from any side effects of fasting, dehydration can even worsen it.

So following liquids/foods should be taken regularly to avoid dehydration.

- 
- Strawberries
- Cantaloupe
- Peaches
- Oranges
- Skim milk
- Lettuce
- Cucumber
- Celery
- Tomatoes
- Plain yogurt
- Water
- Sparkling water
- Black coffee or tea
- Watermelon

All of the above foods are enriched with water and juices. They help the body to fight against dehydration and keep you active and fresh even during fasting hours.

## ✓ Foods For a healthy gut

A growing belly with a lot of fats is clear proof that shows that your gut wellbeing is the way into your general wellbeing. Your gut is home to billions of microorganisms known as the microbiota. These microscopic organisms influence your gut wellbeing, absorption, and psychological wellness. They may likewise assume an urgent job in numerous constant issues.

In this way, you should deal with those minor bugs in your stomach, particularly when you are on irregular fasting. So if you are trying to lose weight, the most important thing is to take care of your stomach. Eat foods that are good for digestion and thus result in reduced body fats.

Following foods are recommended to take for a good stomach helps and to make the digestion process even better.

- All vegetables (especially fresh/raw fruits and veggies)
- Fermented vegetables
- Kefir
- Kimchi
- Kombucha
- Miso
- Sauerkraut
- Tempeh

In addition to that, all these foods also help in weight reduction and trigger the following processes into your body.

- Decreasing absorption of fat.
- Increasing the excretion of saturated/bad fat through stools.

- Reducing food intake.

So you can control your weight by fasting and eating healthy during the nonfasting hours. To your surprise, only healthy eating can also burn your belly fat, keep you healthy and fresh, and reduce extra pounds. So if you're concerned about weight gain, start eating healthy right away and follow the above instructions.

Now, as I have made it clear, what are the foods that should be taken while practicing intermittent fasting. Now let's move towards the foods that should be avoided while practicing intermittent fasting.

Let's have a look at them.

# 10 Foods to avoid while fasting

As mentioned earlier, there is no use of fasting if you are not maintaining a healthy diet. Eating junk or oily foods and ignoring healthy meals might lead you towards different health problems. Doctors and health experts all over the world recommended maintaining a balanced and healthy diet even in non-fasting hours. Eating healthy can help in weight reduction; similarly, eating refined foods can kill the purpose of fasting and results in weight gain and obesity.

The following are the 11 foods that should be avoided if you are practicing intermittent or any other kind of fasting. Let's have a look at them.

## ✗ High added Sugar foods:

White sugar or added sugar is probably the worst thing in our diet these days. Even a spoon of white sugar that you add in a cup of tea is harmful to your heart health and even results in weight reduction and other problems, including cholesterol. Foods high in added sugar usually provide tons of empty calories but are not very filling.

Examples of foods that may contain massive amounts of added sugar include sugary breakfast cereals, granola bars, and low-fat, flavored yogurt. You should be especially careful when selecting "low-fat" or "fat-free" foods, as manufacturers often add lots of sugar to make up for the flavor that's lost when the fat is removed.

High amounts of sugar are present in container juices, fruits, and especially in baked items like cakes, pastries, donuts, ice creams, and the list is long. So if you are practicing fasting and your main purpose of fasting is to reduce some extra pounds, say no to high added sugar foods and stick with your decision.

There is one simple technique to avoid sugary foods. "Move your head left and right, whenever someone offers you processed food."

## ✖ High-calorie Coffee:

Coffee is enriched in caffeine, which is a high level of the biologically active substance. Though it is recommended to take a cup or half of the black coffee while fasting, overdose caffeine is recommended at all. As during fasting, our body is running low on calories and energy levels. We are cutting off some extra amount of calories, and in such situations, intake of high-calorie coffee or caffeine might hurt the stomach, or in some cases, caffeine directly affects heartbeat rate as well. Though caffeine is considered as one of the best substances that can improve metabolism and helps in fats reduction, this is a short term result. In longer-term results, we can see several disadvantages of high-calorie coffee on health like nausea, irregular sleep patterns, and disturbed bowel movement. The negative impacts of including undesirable fixings like counterfeit cream and sugar exceed these constructive outcomes of coffee.

Fatty espresso drinks are quite superior to pop. They're stacked with a void/empty calories that are equivalent heavy as a full-fledged dinner. In case you like coffee, it's ideal for adhering to plain, dark espresso when attempting to get in shape. Including a little cream or milk is fine as well. Simply abstain from including sugar, fatty flavors, and other unfortunate fixings.

## ✖ Pizza:

All of us love fast food, especially pizza. One heavy loaded with lots of chicken, olives, and cheese. No one can resist pizza, but you have to control yourself if you are fasting. Pizza is one high calorie baked food that can result in quick weight gain like all other fast foods. The most dangerous thing in pizza is processed meat and heavy amounts of flour. Both of them are high in calories and kill the purpose of fasting. If you are a pizza lover, then try to make 1, 2 slices at home with homemade ingredients like boiled chicken and some fresh vegetables along with the black paper. Home Sauces are also healthier and have lesser calories.

## ✗ Ice-cream:

Ice-cream is unimaginably tasty, yet extremely undesirable. It is high in calories, and most sorts are stacked with sugar. I know no one can resist ice-cream, but it is important to avoid it if you want to lose weight quickly. A little segment of ice cream is fine once in a while, yet the issue is that it's extremely simple to expend huge sums at a time.

Consider making your dessert, utilizing less sugar, and more beneficial fixings like full-fat yogurt and natural products. Likewise, serve yourself a little bit and put the dessert away so you won't wind up eating excessively.

## ✗ Alcohol

Do you know that alcohol provides a greater number of calories as compared to carbs and proteins? Alcohol provides seven calories per gram that indicate one glass of alcohol is enriched with hundreds of calories that can influence your weight loss journey. Though the evidence of alcohol and its effects on weight reductions are not clear, the intake of high-calorie drinks might affect it negatively. In addition to that, as all of us already know that alcohol is hazardous to health, an overdose of it has many harmful effects on human health. A normal dose of alcohol is fine, but an overdose of alcohol results in weight gain and will also kill the main purpose of fasting, i.e., "healthy lifestyle."

The type of alcohol you are drinking also matters a lot, if you are having a beer, it might not be good for weight loss, but wine is okay with your weight loss journey as well.

## ✖ Cakes and Cookies:

Baked items like cakes, pastries, donuts, candies, and cookies are not at all recommended during your fasting routines. All Of these things are enriched with white added sugar and refined flour that is very hazardous for health and might result in some diseases like diabetes. In addition to that, they also consist of trans fats, and health experts suggest avoiding those fats during fasting practice. Pastries and cakes have fake calories, and once you have them, you will feel hungry again after a few hours. Pieces of candy are very unhealthy as well. They pack a ton of added white sugar, including oils and refined flour, into a little bundle.

Pieces of candy are high in calories and low in supplements. A normally measured piece of candy shrouded in chocolate can contain around 200–300 calories, and extra-huge bars may contain considerably progressively

Shockingly, you can discover sweet treats all over. They are even deliberately submitted in stores in request to entice buyers into getting them incautiously.

If you are craving something sweet, it is better to put your hands on some fruits or eat nuts instead.

If you have a sweet tooth and you usually crave sweets, it is better to make a piece of dark chocolate for yourself.

## ✗ Processed juices:

Many juices that you might find on the shelves of the superstore are not juices at all. Instead, they are artificial flavors with a lot of added sugars. The juice is nothing but just fraud in the name of fruits and vegetables. Natural product juices are exceptionally prepared and stacked with sugar. Indeed, they can contain the same amount of sugar and calories as pop, if not increase. Processed juices are one of the biggest reasons for obesity around the world, especially in children. They fall for the flavor and packaging every time without knowing what's inside the box. Every parent must restrict their kids from adding sugar foods. Otherwise, they have to deal with the consequences.

Likewise, natural product squeeze generally has no fiber and doesn't require biting. This implies a glass of squeezed orange won't have indistinguishable consequences for totality from an orange, making it simple to devour enormous amounts in a short measure of time. Avoid natural product juices and eat the entire organic products instead.

## ✘ White bread:

White bread is part of our everyday groceries. Almost all of us buy it on a daily or sometimes weekly basis without knowing the fact that white bread is enriched with refined flour and a lot of added sugar. White bread is one of the main causes of obesity in many individuals. In addition to that, it is high on the glycemic index that can spike your blood sugar levels at once. According to a study conducted on 1000 people, it is indicated that even two slices of white bread results in a 40% higher risk of weight gain and obesity.

If you love bread, it's okay to replace your white bread with brown bread, which is relatively better and low on calories.

Many people, during their fasting hours, eat a slice or half of the bread, considering it as a light eatable to regain their energy. It is very wrong if You want to lose weight with the help of fasting and refrain from eating white bread right away.

## ✖ Sugary drinks

High sugary drinks like soda, cocktails, soft drinks, coke, and colas are the unhealthiest things that are currently present on the face of the planet. These sugary soft drinks are directly related to weight gain and also results in many other health hazards if consumed daily. Though these sugary drinks consist of hundreds of calories, they don't provide energy to your body. Instead, their only contribution is towards weight gain and disease like diabetes. If you are serious about your weight loss and want to get great benefit out of fasting, then is the time to goodbye to all these fancy drinks. Instead, drink fresh juices if you can't control your cravings.

## ✖ Fried potatoes chips:

Who doesn't fall for a pack full of fries? I know every one of us is fans of French fries and can't avoid them, once they are in front of us. That because we don't know about the contribution of fried chips towards weight gain and obesity. French fries are directly related to obesity, especially in kids and teenagers. Although potatoes are filling and healthy, but not fries. Fries are oily and high in calories. In addition to that, they are light on the stomach, and that's why we usually end up eating a lot of potato chips. One research found that potato chips may contribute to more weight gain per serving than any other food present on this planet. Also, processed, simmered, or fried potatoes may contain cancer-causing substances called acrylamides. Consequently, it's ideal for eating plain or boiled potatoes instead. Precisely, if you want no hindrance in your weight loss journey, now is the time to say goodbye to potato chips.

Reducing weight and maintaining good health is not easy. It requires a lot of effort and hard work. One of the hardest things, it demands is to restrict your food choices. Avoid all the unhealthy and junk you are taking in life and replace it with health, fresh, and home-cooked food. Managing your healthy diet is one of the best ways to reduce weight, and that also is the only purpose of fasting.

# Meal Plans to follow while fasting:

As in intermittent fasting, you are allowed to take 500-600 calories during fasting hours and days. 500 calories are idle for women, and 600 calories are good for men, on the other hand. During fasting hours, we must need some foods that are filling, healthy, and very low on calories at the same time. It is better to pre-planned your diet for fasting things. Deciding what to eat and what not to eat in fasting hours is surely a tough thing. But here I have tried to sort it out for you all. The following are some low on calories yet filling and very healthy diet plans for you all. Let's have a look at it.

## Plan 1:

For Breakfast: Quaker Oats mini sachet of porridge (40g) -that has an estimated 255 calories.

For Dinner: Beetroot and feta salad estimated 125 calories

Beetroot (50g) 13 calories, feta (30g) 83 calories, spinach (60g) 29 calories, A squeeze of lemon 0 calories, Sliced apple with 1 tbsp. of almond butter - 145 could be taken as Snacks. The total calorie count of this diet meal plan is about 525 calories that are idle to take on fasting days.

## Plan 2:

For Breakfast:

- take Sweet plums along with yogurt estimated 145 calories
- 100g low-fat natural yogurt estimated 65 calories
- And two plums - 60 calories
- 1 tsp. of honey - 20 calories

For Dinner:

- Take Ryvita and tuna slices - 253 calories
- Two original Ryvita cracker pieces of bread - 70 calories
- tuna mayo (60g) - 171 calories
- rocket (70g) sprinkled on top - 12 calories
- cracked black pepper - 0 calories

For Snack:

- Miso soup - 32 calories

The total calorie count of the above diet meal plan is 430 calories that are idle to maintain your energy during fasting days.

# Plan 3:

For Breakfast: Packet of Belvita Breakfast Biscuits estimated 228 calories

For Dinner: Roasted vegetables along with balsamic glaze estimated 261 calories

- ½ courgette, ½ aubergine, ½ butternut squash, ½ red pepper estimated 247 calories
- 1 tbsp. balsamic vinegar - 14 calories
- A squeeze of lemon - 0 calories

For Snack:

- Harley's without sugar jelly pot - 4 calories

The total calorie count is round about 493 calories per meal. This meal plan is excellent to take in fasting days to resume your energy and stay active during fasting hours. Let's move towards plan no four now.

# Plan 4:

For Breakfast: take Soft boiled egg1 only) and asparagus estimated 90 calories

- One egg - 70 calories
- Five pieces of asparagus - 20 calories
- salt and pepper to season (it's optional though)

For Dinner: Turkey burgers with corns estimated 328 calories

- turkey mince that is beaten along with small egg
- spring onion,
- garlic and chili (111g)
- Some corns 56 calories

For Snack:

- A few frozen grapes - 60 calories

The total calorie count of this meal plan is 478 calories, and it is one of the light, fulfilling, and healthy diet plans suitable to every individual. You can take it while fasting days and keep yourself fresh and healthy.

## Plan 5:

For Breakfast: take Banana and low-fat yogurt that has an estimated 177 calories.

- 100g low-fat natural yogurt - 65 calories
- One banana - 112 calories
- A sprinkle of cinnamon - no calories

For Dinner: take Turkey breasts with wilted spinach. It has an estimated 216 calories.

- One turkey breast steak (125g) - 175 calories

- 1 cup of spinach that is cooked and seasoned along with salt (according to your taste) - 41 calories

For Snack: take 10g of popcorn. a very healthy yet light snack that has many health benefits with approximately 59 calories

The total calorie count of this diet meal plan is 452 calories, enough to give you energy during fasting days.

## Plan 6:

For Breakfast: spinach omelet, one of my favorite breakfasts that has estimate 160calories.

- Two eggs 140 calories
- spinach leaves (60g) - 20 calories
- salt and pepper according to your taste they have no calories

For Dinner: take Hummus and crudités consist of 175 calories approximately.

- hummus (40g) - 123 calories
- a medium bowl full of carrots, cucumber, raw pepper or any other raw fruit or vegetable - 52 calories

For Snack: Edamame beans (60g) and rock salt - 84 calories

The total calorie count of this meal plan is 419 calories best for both men and women.

## Plan 7:

This is my favorite and most tasty meal diet plan for fasting days.

For Breakfast: you can have Apple, carrot and ginger smoothie with counted 107 calories

- 1 apple - 55 calories

- 1 carrot - 52

- raw ginger - no calories

For Dinner: the most delicious, filling and healthy Pitta pizza - 178 calories

- 25g Extra Light Philadelphia cheese - 40 calories

- 1 tomato - 32 calories

- mixed herbs (as you wish) - no calories

- salt and pepper (according to your taste) - no calories

For Snack: 100g blueberries and some almonds- 137 calories

The total calorie count of this meal plan is 422 calories.

# Plan 8:

For Breakfast: take 2-3Blueberry Buttermilk Pancakes. It has a calorie count of 206 calories

For Dinner: you can have Roasted red pepper along with tomato soup with cracker breads - 128 calories

- 2 original Ryvita cracker pieces of bread - 70 calories
- ½ red pepper, ½ tomato, ½ onion, garlic clove, 1 tsp. tomato puree, ½ tsp. cumin, Oxo chicken, stock cube, ½ tsp. balsamic vinegar, salt (as your wish) and some seasonal herbs (according to your taste).

For Snack: 1 tbsp. of pumpkin and sunflower seeds, whichever you like the most. Both these seeds are good for health and low on calories. Both combined have 90 calories approximately.

The total calorie count of this meal plan is 424 calories.

# Plan 9:

For Breakfast: take one full (average size) Mixed berry bowl that has 115 calories. You can take following berries to fill up the bowl

- strawberries (100g) - 30 calories
- raspberries - (100g) - 28 calories
- blueberries - (100g) - 57 calories

For Dinner: take Harissa chicken with grilled vegetables - 314 calories

- 1 chicken breast (130g) - 160 calories
- 100g of vegetable - 139 calories
- 1 tbsp. harissa paste - 15 calories

For Snack: Pistachios (around 10-12) - 60 calories

The total calorie count of this meal plan is 489 calories. This is one of my favorite and tasty meal diet plans. That is good for your health as well as it soothes your taste buds too.

## Plan 10:

For Breakfast: you can have some of your favorite fruit and nut muesli (50g) that has 190 calories

For Dinner: take Pesto salmon with curly kale - 293 calories

- salmon fillet (100g) - 180 calories
- 3 tsp. of green pesto- 80 calories
- steamed kale with a reasonable amount of black pepper (100g) - 33 calories

For snacks: 60g of stoned cherries - 23 calories

The total calorie count is 506 calories

So here are 10best meal plans that are good to have on your fasting days. You can select the one that you liked the most or change them according to your requirements and food cravings. All of the above meat plans are filling, healthy, and very low on calories. None of the above is more than 600 calories, and that's the best thing about all these diet plans.

The purpose of creating the low-calorie meet plan for you all is to make fasting an easy thing for you. If you think fasting means to give up on all your favorite food, then you might be wrong.

**The main purpose of fasting is to lose weight and maintain good body health.** The following are the 15 best foods that are "most weight loss-friendly foods" currently present on the face of this planet.

Let's talk about them:

# 15 best Weight-friendly Foods:

Different foods have different counts of calories and energy. Some foods are weight loss-friendly foods, whereas some result in sudden weight gain, and that's why we need to find out some foods that are filling, healthy, low on calories, and helps in weight loss reduction. The following 15 foods are healthy yet effective in reducing some extra pounds.

## Yogurt:

Dairy products are enriched in calcium that makes your bones strong and healthy. On the other hand, they have a lot of filling and healthy calories that keep you fresh and active all day. Yogurt is one healthy dairy product with lots of calcium and probiotics that helps in keeping your stomach healthy and improves its function. A healthy stomach results in a better digestion process, hence; help towards an individual's weight loss journey. Also, try to take full-fat yogurt, full-fat yogurt helps in weight reduction as well as it prevents body against diseases like type 2 diabetes. Processed or low-fat yogurt that usually comes in containers high on added sugar, that's why I wouldn't recommend it to you.

Make full-fat yogurt a part of your daily diet, and in a few weeks, you will see good results.

## Whole Eggs:

Eating a lot of eggs produced bad LDL cholesterol, and that's why it is dangerous for people to have some heart diseases or to suffer from cholesterol already. But eggs are a very filling, healthy, and nutritious diet for the people who are trying hard to lose weight. Some studies and research have shown that people who take at least two eggs in breakfast stay active the whole day, and they don't feel fatigued or laziness for the next 36 hours. Eggs are enriched with protein and fats that help in weight reduction without affecting muscle mass.

The egg yolk is enriched with all the nutrition. I would recommend you to take boiled eggs rather than fried or whisked one.

## Coconut oil:

All fats are not created equal; they get dissolved in the body and results in different calories count. Coconut oil consists up of high fatty acid that of medium length. Researchers have shown that these high fatty acids result in better burning of stored calories that help in weight loss and belly fat reduction. In addition to that, fatty acids are filling and give a lot of energy to the body.

Two different studies conducted on men and women separately show that coconut oil is good for belly fat reduction.

Adding coconut oil to some of the other foods is not recommended. That's because it is calorie enriched and doesn't make a good combination with other foods. Instead, it's a better idea to replace your normal cooking oil with coconut oil.

In addition to that, extra virgin oil is one of the healthiest and fat reducing oil on this planet currently.

## Chia seeds:

Chia seeds are one of the most fiber-containing food. It is one of the healthiest foods that give the body adequate energy and keeps it healthy. One gram of chia seeds has 12 calories, but don't worry 11 of these calories are fiber, and the remaining one is carbs. So this low on carbs and high fiber food are best for weight reduction in burning fats. It also helps in better gut health and improves hormonal problems in women also.

Some researchers have revealed that taking one teaspoon of chia seeds every day also helps in the better menstrual cycle and thus helps in weight reduction. Dropped or irregular periods are one of the biggest causes of obesity in women.

Chia seeds, in some cases, also result in lost appetite. Less appetite means you will have fewer suppers that will directly affect the body's weight.

## Grapefruit:

Though all the fresh fruits are good for a healthy body and mind, citrus fruits above all are one of the best fruits that helps in weight loss. But here, highlighting grapefruit is quite important. Studies and researches have shown the direct impact of grapefruit on the body's weight reduction. According to a study conducted on 90 obese people, it has been stated that eating grapefruits before any meal for 12 weeks can result in weight loss (3.5 pounds approximately).

Researchers have shown grapefruit contribution towards insulin resistance and metabolic disturbance that can further lead the body towards many other chronic diseases like type 2 diabetes.

All you need to do is just eat some grapefruit, approximately half an hour before every meal, and then see the results in just a few weeks. Grapefruit is one of the best foods that is filling, healthy, and helps in belly fat reduction.

## Fruits and Vegetables

Fresh fruits and veggies are the best combinations of all the important minerals, calcium, protein, and fibers that you should take in your daily meals. All fruits and vegetables are enriched with a lot of vitamins that keep you not only healthy but also very active and prevent your body against all the effects. I suggest you, every day may be in your lunch, and prepare a separate place of raw fruits and vegetables.

Cut them down (half a plate of fruits and another half of veggies) and eat it as it is. The more colors you add to the plate, the more vitamins and nutrition you will intake.

Fruits and vegetables not only are healthy diets, but eating them raw also helps in belly fat reduction and keeps you active all day.

## Nuts:

As soon as we hear the word "nuts," the first thing that comes up in our minds is one fattening food. Though nuts are high in calories, they are not as fattening as you think. They are one of the healthiest snacks on the face of the planet that are enriched with protein, fiber, and a lot of healthy fats. Nuts are filling and healthy and also results in weight reduction. Even eating a handful of nuts gives you a feeling of a full stomach, and you won't eat meals for longer periods.

Researches have shown that nuts are good for improved metabolism and belly fat reduction. In addition to that, it has been proved; people who eat nuts daily have healthier bodies as compared to those who don't.

But do not overdose, a handful of nuts is enough for one day.

## Apple Vinegar:

Apple vinegar is one of the best things that helps in weight reduction. You can add iron in regular foods like salads and fruits, or some people just take it with water and drink a glass of water or juice mixed with several drops of apple vinegar. A few human-based examinations propose that apple juice vinegar can be helpful for weight reduction.

Taking vinegar simultaneously as a high-carb feast can expand sentiments of totality and cause individuals to eat 200–275 fewer calories for the remainder of the day

One 12-week concentrate on corpulent people additionally demonstrated that 15 or 30 ml of vinegar for every day caused a weight reduction of 2.6–3.7 pounds, or 1.2–1.7 kilograms

Vinegar has likewise been appeared to diminish glucose spikes after dinners, which may have different useful and healthy impacts on human health.

## Avocados:

Avocado is one of the healthiest and unique fruits. It has millions of health benefits and also a great fruit to eat during your weight loss journey. Avocados are enriched in monounsaturated oleic acid. These similar acids are found in olive oil as well. Though avocados consist of a lot of fats, it is not at all a fattening food. They are enriched with a lot of water and fibers that are great for belly fat reduction and helps maintain the best health.

Avocados are one of the best foods for pregnant women as well. They prevent morning sickness and help maintain body health and water level. Also, they're an ideal expansion to vegetable servings of mixed greens, as studies show that their fat substance can expand carotenoid cancer prevention agents; they additionally contain numerous significant supplements, including fiber and potassium.

Avocados are a genuine case of a solid fat source you can remember for your eating regimen while attempting to get in shape. Simply make a point to keep your avocado's intake adequate.

## Water:

Having a healthy and perfect body has a price. And this price is to ignore all the fancy drinks, cocktails and sugary juices. Instead, try to drink a lot of water. Though water is not food, it is an essential part of all the foods. Fruits, veggies, meats, and even the human body is 97% water already. It means water is an essential drink that is important to keep your organs healthy. Drinking a lot of water prevents kidney disease. It purifies your blood and results in glowing and fresh skin.

14 glasses of water every day are ideal for human consumption. In addition to that drinking, a lot of water helps in weight reduction as well. As it detoxifies the body and helps to maintain the body's health

## Health benefits of fasting:

Fasting has several health benefits for human health. The one above all is weight reduction and burning extra stored body fats that can lead you towards many diseases. Let's talk about fasting and its impact on human health.

# Promotes detoxification:

Another great advantage of fasting is that it advances the detoxification of the body.

A significant number of the prepared nourishments we eat today contain bunches of added substances, some of which are poisonous to our bodies. As the nourishment is processed and ingested into the body, these poisons are likewise retained into the body and put away in fat stores around the body. During fasting, your mind regards the nourishing hardship as a danger and responds by initiating versatile pressure reactions to assist it with managing the risk. The brain additionally begins examining how it will give the body energy without nourishment. To guarantee that the metabolism is still working in its optimal condition, the brain then triggers the transformation of glycogen that is stored in the body and starts converting it into energy packets.

Although glycogen is not very healthy for the body and energy produced by it is not so useful, after the 12 hours of fasting, the glycogen deposits get depleted. Now, the body must locate another option for energy. As the fat stores are signed to give energy, the poisons put away inside the fats are discharged. These poisons are then expelled from the body with the assistance of the liver, kidneys, and different organs, leaving your body liberated from gathered poisons.

## Fights Inflammation

According to some research done, chronic inflammation can lead the human body towards dangerous diseases, including heart disease, some types of cancer, and arthritis. Fasting helps the human body to fight against chronic inflammation. A study was conducted having 15 adults fasting for a few days, resulting in having fewer levels of body inflammation.

Though inflammation has a lot of health benefits, it prevents the body against certain diseases, but at the same time, acute inflammation can lead to serious health consequences. We can say that fasting helps in the reduction of inflammation, thus provokes a healthy lifestyle.

## A fresh and healthy skin:

If you are using different vanishing and beauty creams to make your skin better and free of acne, you might be doing it wrong. To your surprise, fasting is one of the best ways to make skin lighter, clearer, and more healthy-looking. As we have discussed earlier, that fasting helps in cleaning and detoxification, so as a result, we get clear and poison-free skin. At the point when you are fasting, your body recovers the cells that make up your skin and cleans old cell material from existing cells, in this way adding to a superior look. This recovery can even add to the mending of scars. Especially acne scars. We likewise observed that fasting diminishes irritation and inflammation, which is one of the biggest reasons for some skin conditions like skin inflammation, acne, scars, and uneven skin tone. Improving how your skin looks, fasting additionally helps to sound and solid hair and nails and brightens your eyes.

With everything taken into account, fasting not just improves how you feel; it likewise improves what you look like.

## Better heart Health

According to a survey, heart diseases are one of the major causes of death around the globe. Heart attacks due to thinning of veins and arteries, high cholesterol levels in the blood are the few major heart diseases. Fasting helps a lot in making your heart strong and healthy. A healthy body must have a healthy heart. Healthy fasting hours contribute a lot to heart health and help your heart to perform in better ways. One survey showed that two months of alternate-day fasting decreased degrees of LDL cholesterol and blood triglycerides by 25% and 32% individually. It means fasting is highly helpful in reducing the bad cholesterol level in the blood and purifies the blood as well.

## Weight loss:

A large number of individuals who are doing fasting are doing it to have a healthy body. Of course, a healthy lifestyle is only the purpose of fasting. A healthy body has a healthy mind. So fasting contributes towards both a healthy mind and a healthy body. A healthy body means to maintain your body weight. A healthy body doesn't have a few pounds and nor it has 100 above pounds. To maintain your weight, it is important to take a healthy diet, and along with that, fasting also helps in weight reduction. When you fast for a few hours, it could be 8, 10,12, 16,24, or sometimes 48 hours; your body starts burning stored fats and hence results in weight reduction. The best thing about fasting is, it is helpful in weight loss without affecting muscle mass. Moreover, irregular fasting upgrades hormone capacity to encourage weight reduction.

Lower insulin levels, higher development hormone levels, and expanded measures of norepinephrine (noradrenaline) all expand the breakdown of muscle to fat ratio and encourage its utilization for vitality. So precisely, we can say that fasting builds your metabolic rate by 3.6-14% and helps in belly reduction. At the end of the day, intermittent fasting chips away at the two sides of the calorie condition.

## Better Nervous System:

Not only body but fasting has a lot of healthy impact on brain cells and its activities as well. According to research that is mainly conducted on animals, it has been seen that fasting helps in recovering brain cells and to improve the nervous system of the body. Intermittent fasting for 11 months or more can improve both brain cells and brain structure. Fasting also helps in better cognitive systems by producing more nerve cells.

## Better sleeping routine:

According to some research, it is stated that fasting has a direct impact on your sleep patterns, and it helps to give you better sleep at night. It is stated that a person who is fasting for several weeks would fall asleep quickly, and he will wake up fresher and more active. It is suggested that a human should take his last meal a few hours before sleeping. Because the digestion process works best when you are awake and active. Once you lay down in your bed, the digestion becomes slower.

## Controlled blood sugar:

According to some recent research that includes ten individuals with type-2 diabetes demonstrated that transient irregular fasting altogether diminished glucose levels in the blood and regulated the amount of insulin it. Moving on, another audit found that both alternate-day fasting and 24 hours fasting was as successful as constraining calorie consumption at lessening insulin obstruction.

So your body has a lower risk of diabetes, and it has a more regulated amount of sugar in the blood. Combined with the potential glucose bringing down impacts of fasting, this could help keep your glucose consistent, forestalling spikes and crashes in your glucose levels.

## Better Life span:

A healthy lifestyle and healthy body lead towards a longer life span that is also free from diseases and chronic illness. Different researches and studies have shown that people who do fasting have a longer life span as compared to one who doesn't fast. Many types of research have been conducted on animal bodies that show fasting can result in a longer life span and decrease all the aging effects. It includes aged diseases and a lot of other problems. Fasting is like a filter that filters away all the negative and harmful effects from your body, leaving it all fresh and healthy.

# Potential Side-effect of fasting:

Even though we can't overlook the way that irregular fasting has a lot of medical advantages. The previously mentioned are only a couple of them. There are significantly more favorable circumstances that are extraordinary for the human body and increment the life expectancy of people too. There are likewise some negative effects of fasting. Any individual who is going to begin irregular fasting at any point shortly has to know both the positive and negative effects of fasting and afterward choose either its advantageous for your body or not.

## Low sugar level:

If you are diabetic and want to start intermittent fasting, then it is very important to select the right method for it. Otherwise, your body might just throw up, and you might collapse at any time of day. It is recommended to take some low fat and less sugary juices during fasting hours to keep blood sugar level normal. Or you can simply add half a spoon of brown sugar in water with a pinch of salt and drink it once a day. It gives the body a certain amount of sugar and helps you to sustain the fast without body collapse.

## Hair loss:

Human hair needs a lot of vitamins and zinc. The deficiency of vitamin D and zinc might be one of the causes of hair loss. If you see that more hair is falling off during your shower, it means your body needs of nutrition are not fulfilled properly, and you need to stop fasting right now. Or one other way is to start taking multivitamin supplements. So if you are fasting for longer hours it is important to keep multivitamins with you. Multi-vitamins help to restore the body's energy and fulfill its nutritional need.

## Disturbed cycle in women:

You might feel a change in your menstrual cycle. It happens when a woman loses a huge amount of weight at once and not getting the proper calories and nutrition. It might result in changed or disturbed period cycles. According to some research's women with very smart weak bodies suffer from a situation that is commonly known as "Amenorrhea " that's a disease in which either period slows down, or they get completely stopped. Sudden weight loss might disturb your hormones and genes. It might result in other period-related problems like facial hair growth or body pains, especially backaches and leg pain. All of these things happen because of nothing but weakness and an insufficient number of vitamins, nutrition, and proteins in the body.

If you feel any of the above symptoms (changed or stopped period), stop fasting right away, and consult your health expert.


Weight reduction is important, but losing too much weight suddenly might negatively affect you. That's why it is important to keep balance and try to reduce weight through proper steps.

# Physiological effects of fasting:

Though fasting is safe for many healthy individuals. It is reported that fasting improves brain cells' activity and helps in better memory as well. Some people feel extremely good physiological changes have reported in good mood swings. Some researches and studies have shown that fasting for long hours might lead you towards some psychological disorders. Some individuals have reported that all these mood issues get resolved once you get used to the fasting routine. It might be true, but researchers and doctors haven't confirmed this claim yet. Intermittent fasting might trigger your food cravings, and you end up thinking about the food all the time. In addition to that, it might lead you to depression or anxiety. Some times due to lack of energy, people just sit and think all the time. This overthinking is the basic cause of depression and anxiety.

Also, if you already are a depression patient and panics in most situations, itis recommended to concern your health exert before practicing any kind of fasting.

## Hormonal changes:

According to some research, it is said that intermittent fasting might affect the metabolic rate of the body that has a further impact on human hormones. Different individuals have shown different hormonal reactions after intermittent fasting. The studies have shown intermittent fasting is beneficial for some women as it improves fertility. Whereas there are some opposite reactions as well, such as irregular and missed periods and certain kinds of problems that might lead to pregnancy and conceiving complications. Many individuals just focus on how many hours they are fasting and how much weight is lost without paying attention to the nutritious needs of the body. The food we eat is just not calories. It is a composition of vitamins, proteins, calcium, fibers, carbohydrates, and fats. And if you are consuming less nutrition, you may feel laziness, fatigue and might feel hungry all the time, and it will affect your hormones as well.

Make a proper diet plan for non-fasting days and eat healthy meals to properly fulfill your body needs. Different people have different reactions towards fasting, especially women, they might feel greater disadvantages of fasting. If you are feeling any discomfort, stop fasting right away and get the proper medical help.

## Other short term effects of fasting:

- Fatigue
- Dizziness
- Low energy
- Lightheadedness
- Anxiety
- Insomnia
- Extreme hunger
- Low blood sugar

- Constipation

- Fainting

- Irritability

- Hormonal imbalance

- Weight gain

Though I do not deny fasting and its health benefits, if not done properly, fasting might lead you towards the above-mentioned health hazards. I am mentioning it again and again that women should start fasting with medical help. Especially pregnant, breastfeeding women, women trying to conceive or women with weaker immune systems should avoid fasting.

Here is all about fasting and its contribution to health and weight reduction. Fasting is, no doubt, one of the best ways to reduced weight that, too, with a healthy lifestyle. Always remember fasting and healthy eating are inter-connected. If you are ignoring one of these two, you will not get a 10/10 benefit outfit.

## What is Healthy Eating?

Eating a healthy and balanced diet is a crucial part of maintaining good health and helps you to feel better. This leads us to the question of what is healthy eating? The answer is simple, eating a wide range of food in the right proportion and consuming a proper amount of drinks and food to maintain a healthy body. On average, women need to consume 2000 calories, while men are required to consume 2500 calories per day.

There is a famous saying that "Health is wealth"; It means that health is everything. For instance, if one is healthy enough, he can live his life the way he wants. Now, health has got a direct relation to adequate nutrition. By adequate nutrition, we mean such sort of food, which maintains our body fit and functioning well. It protects us from different kinds of diseases and stresses. It is said that if somebody eats junk food, medicine is of no use, and if it is a balanced diet, then there is no need for medication. Thus, healthy food contains such kind of nutrients and carbohydrates, which help us to keep fit both mentally and physically.

Similarly, it is, somehow, relative; everyone has their scale of healthy food, and there is no universal measurement of healthy food. However, vegetables and fresh fruits are considered to be healthy food. Vegetables consist of vitamins(A&C) and minerals, which keep us healthy. It prevents us from diseases like cancer, diabetes, and cardiovascular diseases. Therefore, a balanced diet is critical for our physical, mental, and emotional health.

On the other hand, an imbalanced diet- which is also called junk food- leads to poor health, anxiety, and stress. There are certain foods which are eaten daily, but it can't be considered healthy, for example, fast-food. It has more amount of sugar, salt, and oil, which makes us unhealthy. It also causes obesity and increases the risk of a heart attack.

Healthy dieting doesn't need to be excessively complicated. On the off chance that you feel overwhelmed by all the clashing advice and diet patterns out there, you are not the only one in this confusion. It appears that for each expert who reveals to you a specific nourishment is beneficial for you, you will discover another maxim precisely the inverse. In all actuality, while some particular nourishments or supplements have been appeared to affect temperament beneficially, it's your general dietary example that is generally significant. The foundation of a solid eating routine ought to be to supplant processed food with natural fresh food at whatever point conceivable. Eating nourishment that is as close as credible to nature can make a big difference in how you think, look, and feel. Try to keep your goals modest, and aim for one target at a time. This strategy will surely help you in the long run, if followed accurately.

During fasting, it is immensely vital to eat healthily and maintain the energy levels of the body. It has been observed that many people, especially women, tend to skip breakfast. This can affect the body negatively. Therefore, it is recommended not to skip *breakfast* and eat as per the body's need.

Following are some of the key points for a healthy eating

- Try to eat a variety of food
- Increase the number of fresh fruits and vegetables in your food
- Make sure to eat enough protein
- Reduce the intake of sugar and salt
- Drink plenty of fluid, especially before meals
- Exercise regularly
- Try to avoid processed and packaged food and eat real food
- Don't skip Breakfast

We must be cautious about the selection of food. If we go with the desires and eat whatever is on the table, it may lead to some severe consequences. Usually, very few people pay attention to healthy food and eat whatever they are served with. For the sake of temporary taste, many people eat junk food in abundance, which effects their health negatively. One must be very careful about the selection of food we eat as it is directly related to our mental and emotional health.

Researches show that our mood swings are often dependent on the selection of food. How often have you noticed that we are trying to feed our feelings rather than our bodies? Sometimes human attitudes are directed by unconscious emotions. The food we eat is a practical example of this. Likewise, taking a proper diet can impact our behaviors positively. A good meal changes our mood and increases the efficiency of the body. We feel fresh, energetic, and active.

## Eating Vegetables and Fruits

The vegetables and fruits are a good source of vitamins and minerals. Doctors recommend plant-based eastings more than anything else. An eating rich in vegetables and fresh fruits can bring down blood pressure, lessen the danger of coronary illness and stroke, forestall a few sorts of disease, lower the risk of eye and stomach related issues, and have a positive impact upon blood sugar, which can help hold hunger under control. Apart from that, eating non-starchy fruits and vegetables like apples, pears, and green leafy vegetables may even promote weight reduction.

Surveys show that eating fresh vegetables and fruits reduce the risk of some types of cancer, diabetes, and eyes related diseases. Moreover, it keeps the skin smooth and bright, improves your vision, and leads to a better digestive system.

## Pulses and Healthy Food

Pulses are an essential part of a properly balanced diet and have been appeared to have significant importance in forestalling diseases, for instance, cancer, diabetes, and coronary illness. Pulses are a very rich source of protein and high fiber content.

Pulses are high in fiber, containing both solvent and insoluble fibers. Solvent fiber assists with diminishing blood cholesterol levels and control blood sugar levels, and insoluble fiber assists with digestion.

The World Health Organization evaluates that up to 80% of coronary illness, stroke, and type 2 diabetes and over 33% of tumors could be forestalled by disposing of hazard factors, for example, undesirable eating regimens and advancing better dietary patterns, of which pulses are a fundamental component.

## Milk and Dairy Products

Milk is complete nourishment in macronutrients. Cheese is a top-notch option in contrast to meat, one of which is wealthy in proteins of high biological worth. It is critical to be a part of our daily diet. It is recommended that adults should consume at least one glass of milk daily. Milk, yogurt, and cheese are core aspects of healthy eating patterns and suggested by many international dietary guidance organizations.

## Dry Fruits and its Impacts on Health

Almost all dry fruits are rich in proteins, minerals, vitamins, and fiber. Additionally, they are delicious and tasty as well. It could be an excellent substitute for daily snacks. It improves the stamina and maintains the energy levels of the body. Dry fruits are a rich source of fiber, which means better digestion and health. Apart from that, dry fruits contain protein, calcium, copper, iron, potassium, magnesium, zinc, riboflavin, phosphorus, and vitamin A-C-E-K-B6. It means healthy skin, teeth, bones, nerves, and muscles. This also means protection from cardiovascular diseases, anemia, high cholesterol, and strengthening of the immune system.

## Reducing the quantity of Sugar and Salt

Consuming too much sugar affects your health adversely. The high intake of sugar may lead to some severe aftermaths. One of the most common problems is faced by those who intake sugar in abundance is obesity, diabetes, and cardiovascular diseases. Similarly, the high intake of salt results in high blood pressure, which increases the possibility of a heart attack. Added sugar, salt, and fats are found in abundance in canned foods, fast foods, beverages, soft drinks, and many more. So, the question is, what can you actually do to avoid or reduce the consumption of sugar, salt, and fats? The answer is simple. Try to replace processed food with natural fresh food. It seems difficult, but once you get to it, you will comfortable and satisfied. If you are opting for more natural and fresh foods, it will surely affect positively the way you see, think, and feel.

## Healthy Breakfast

Undoubtedly, Breakfast is the most significant feast of the day; however, do any of us know why? Other than the way that morning meal diets are hands-down better than the other two meals of the day, your body benefits when you snatch some grub before you head off to begin your day. Studies have indicated that gobbling not long after you wake up can help give your digestion a lift, which can diminish levels of yearning later in the day, fend off weakness, and give you additional vitality throughout the day.

Breakfast propensities can bolster weight reduction; however, how these functions shift from individual to individual. Having breakfast may help weight reduction for certain individuals as they remain full for more time, which forestalls eating during the day. For other people, skipping breakfast bolsters weight reduction since it drives them to devour fewer calories generally.

Shedding pounds requires an individual to consume fewer calories than they eat. To continue weight reduction, an individual must adhere to a diminished calorie diet and pair this eating regimen with greater movement. To roll out supportable dietary improvements, it is fundamental that an individual finds fortifying nourishments they appreciate eating.

Exceptionally prohibitive weight control plans are frequently hard to follow. Rather, fuse a couple of treats and find feeding, low-calorie nourishments that taste great. A dietitian or specialist can enable an individual to build up the correct supper plan for their necessities.

Breakfast is the first and most important of the day. We need to start our day with a healthy breakfast. That is why breakfast is essential. Furthermore, some people skip breakfast, but that could be dangerous. To remain active, fresh, and energetic – breakfast holds a critical role in our dietary patterns. Therefore, we need to start our day with a healthy breakfast.

## Consuming more Water

At the point when the stomach detects that it is full, it imparts signs to the cerebrum to quit eating. Water can assist with occupying room in the stomach, prompting a sentiment of completion and lessening hunger. An individual may likewise believe that they are eager when they are parched. Drink a glass of water before eating can assist with checking excessive eating. Additionally, some studies suggest that consuming more Water can help you to burn calories. It has been observed that drinking more Water increases the melting of fats and helps to lose weight.

## Healthy Eating and its Impacts on Health

One way or another, we all know that our diet impacts our health. Similarly, junk food leads to obesity, which itself is a significant reason for many diseases. On the other hand, healthy food prevents us from many fatal diseases. Eating junk food loaded with fats, sugar, and salt is a major cause of obesity. This burdens the body and organs have to work hard to maintain the functions of the body. Furthermore, it increases the risk of heart diseases, stroke, diabetes, osteoporosis, and several others.

Good health is a blessing of God. To perform the duties to the best of our abilities and live a healthy life, it is of utmost importance to take care of our eating. Healthy eating is just like the fuel of the human body through which we perform our daily based activities. A balanced diet keeps us healthy, strong, and energetic. Eating a variety of food, more vegetables & fruits, consuming 8-10 glass of water and regular exercise are some of the key components which help to keep healthy and live a beautiful life.

## Relationship between healthy eating and weight loss:

The connection between nourishment and health is a difficult one. Everybody needs food to live; however, too little food, a lot of food, or an inappropriate kind of food has negative impacts on health. It is vital to keep an eye on the diet we eat daily. Over 2,500 years back, Hippocrates stated: "Let food be thy medicine and medicine be thy food." Healthy food can optimize both short and long haul health and can help lessen the chance for some health conditions.

The connection between individuals and food is mind-boggling. Food is found in abundance in the United States. The overconsumption of calories is the main factor of the obesity problem. Therefore, obesity is common in the USA. In the United States, food producers spend almost $11 billion in a year for the marketing of these foods. Most of these are not considered healthy, full of sugar, salt, and fat. The main target of marketers is the youth of society. They spend $1.8 billion on the marketing of snack food and high-calorie beverages. Thus, it has resulted in a dramatic increase in these products. Approximately 60% of children's Tv programs advertise food eaten outside of mealtime. 34% of these advertisements are of snacks and candies, followed by soda and other soft drinks with 9%. Apart from that, it also promotes the beauty ideal of dangerously thin, which, as a result, increases eating disorders by continuously taking demands for food that makes it extremely hard to get to the desired weight goals seat by individuals.

Changing your dietary patterns is key to losing and keeping up your weight. To get more fit, you need to eat fewer calories and utilize a higher number of calories than you take in. This can be trying for some individuals to accomplish for an all-inclusive timeframe. Recent studies show that staying with an eating plan might be essential to losing and keeping up weight than the kind of eating plan you follow.

After many studies and researches, it has been found that it is difficult for most people to keep weight off after reducing weight. The reason is simple; people tend to go back to their previous routine and diet. Apart from that, the metabolism also signals you to switch to the old diet. All these factors, when combined, make it hard for the individual to stick to the new diet and reject the motivation for regaining the weight. On the other hand, those who are successful in maintaining their reduced weight have carefully arranged their diet habits, routine, and daily intake of calories and fats. Therefore, by any means, it is not an easy task to maintain weight after reducing it.

A healthy diet plan helps you to manage your weight includes a great variety of food. Try to focus on the following diet plan to eat healthily, and the weight remains under control.

## Eat the Rainbow

One needs to add different varieties and colors of food to its plate. Oranges, tomatoes, leafy greens, and even fresh herbs are a rich source of vitamins, fiber, and minerals. The addition of frozen broccoli, peppers, and onions gives a convenient and quick boost of color and nutrients. Apart from that, you can also add red sauce by using canned tomatoes (No salt added).

## Fresh, Frozen, Dry or Canned Fruits

We must not be obsessed only with bananas and apples only. All fresh and canned fruits can be an excellent choice. Pineapples, mangoes, kiwi fruit, or juice could add more energy and taste to our diet plan. One must be cautious about the canned fruits as it may contain added sugar. However, we must keep an eye on the ingredient list printed on the pack. It is better to go for its natural juice or even water.

## Fresh, Frozen, or Canned Vegetables

Trying some of the fresh, frozen, or even canned vegetables could be a fantastic idea. Besides the health benefits, it could activate our taste buds, and we would have some fantastic tasty foods on the table. As we mentioned above, when it comes to canned vegetables, we should take care of there is no salt added. It is better to avoid salt without added salt. The canned vegetable could be much more beneficial. Additionally, it is really not a bad idea to try something new every week.

# Calcium-Rich Foods

When we say calcium, our mind automatically thinks of a glass of milk and other dairy products. It is quite right, a glass of milk, without sugar, could be a fantastic choice to fulfill the needs of calcium in our body. Furthermore, a bowl of fat-free or low-fat yogurt without sugar, which comes in a variety of different flavors, can be a desirable replacement of a dessert on the table.

# Switching from your Favorite Dish

It is not easy to switch from your favorite dish to arguably a new healthier dish. What about opting for dry beans instead of frying fish or breaded chicken? Beans are a low-fat dish full of vitamins and could be an excellent substitute for other high-fat meat dishes. This is a healthy switch from your favorite dish as it helps to maintain the essential need for vitamins to our bodies.

# What is the Best Way for Healthy Weight-Loss?

If you take any book for diet, and the best foods for reducing weight, they all have elaborated it differently. This is a fact that there is no universal solution to weight loss. Different people have different experiences and results in the same diet. Additionally, it depends on several factors, for example, genetics, climate, and the body's response to various foods. Therefore, the experts are divided upon the best food for the reduction of weight. On the contrary, it has been witnessed that those who work hard, remain consistent, and not afraid of different experimentation get the desired results.

While a few people react well to tallying calories or comparable prohibitive strategies, others react better to having more opportunities in arranging their health improvement plans. If a diet plan has worked for one person, and the same diet does not produce the same results for you, it is absolutely fine, and you do not need to feel degraded. Furthermore, don't thrash yourself if an eating routine demonstrates unreasonably prohibitive for you to stay with. Finally, in all that process, consistency is the key. So, you need to follow that eating routine, which you think you can follow for a longer period.

Even though there is no universal solution to the obesity problem, however, there are several measures you can take to get the maximum results out of it. Try to build up a more beneficial connection with nourishment, check passionate triggers to gorging, and accomplish a healthy weight.

We will discuss the four most effective ways for the reduction of healthy weight.


- Cut Calories
- Cut Carbohydrates

- Cut Fats

- Follow the Mediterranean Diet

## 1. Cut Calories

Many experts admit that effectively dealing with your weight boils down to a primary condition: If you really want to lose weight, you must burn more calories than you take. Sounds simple, correct? At that point, why is losing weight so hard?

Weight reduction is certifiable, not a direct occasion after some time. When you reduce the intake of calories, you may drop weight for the initial barely any weeks, and when some time passes, everything takes a turn. People switch back to their old routine and start taking the same number of calories, which affects the overall performance. As a result, the individual does not achieve their goals. I, once again, would say that taking fewer calories and burning more calories is the most factor in reducing weight.

Besides, all calories are not equal. Some foods contain calories that are more than just a calorie and can affect your body entirely in a different way than the other foods' calories. An essential factor is that we need to opt for foods that are rich in calories yet don't cause you to feel full (like treats) and supplant them with vegetables. Vegetables contain a lot of water and not excessively filled with calories.

Most of us not eat basically to fulfill our hunger. We likewise go to nourishment for comfort or to calm pressure—which can rapidly crash any weight-reduction plan.

## 2. Cut Carbohydrates

Various surveys suggest that the problem is not devouring such a large number of calories, yet instead how the body amasses fat after expending starches— precisely the job of the hormone insulin. At the point when you eat dinner, your body consumes the sugar in the shape of glucose. For that reason, to maintain the level of glucose in the body, the human body regularly extracts glucose from the food we eat.

If you eat a starch-rich feast, for example, the French fries, bread, or rice, it converts into fats. All these foods are rich in carbs, and if you are not up to the task and unable to burn these starch-rich foods, it will surely convert into fats, which is always undesirable. If you do not burn the consumed carbs, as a result, you gain extra weight, and your body now requires more fuel to consume. Hence, you eat more. Since insulin just consumes sugars, you need carbs, thus starts an endless loop of devouring carbs and putting on weight. To lose weight, the thinking goes, you have to break this cycle by diminishing carbs.

Most low-carb slims down supporter supplanting carbs with protein and fat, which could have some negative long haul consequences for your health. Consequently, we must go for low carbs foods as it reduces the danger of its conversion into fats. As an alternate, the green vegetables, especially unprocessed, the dairy item which has low fats, can be an excellent replacement.

## 3. Cut Fats

It's a backbone of numerous eating regimens: on the off chance that you would prefer not to get fat, don't eat fat. Walk down any supermarket passageway, and you will be bombarded with decreased fat snacks, dairy, and packaged foods. Yet, while our low-fat alternatives have detonated, so have obesity rates. This is the prime reason that the mentioned plan has not been so practical for the reduction of weight.

Not all fats are bad. Some fats are actually essential for the body. Good fats are the most important feature of the Mediterranean diet. Such fats can be found abundantly in fish and milk. These fats are termed as good fats or healthy fats. As we all know that milk is beneficial and an integral part of the balanced diet. These fats are unsaturated fats, and the burning of these fats is much easier than saturated fats.

We regularly make an inappropriate exchange offs. A considerable lot of us tragically swap fat for the empty calories of sugar and refined starches. Rather than eating whole-fat yogurt, most of the people switch to foods that are even more dangerous. Therefore, it is critical to arrange our food choices carefully and make such a replacement are both healthy and low on bad fats.

## 4. Follow the Mediterranean Diet

The Mediterranean eating routine stresses eating "good" fats and carbs alongside vast amounts of green vegetables, fresh fruits, and cheese. The Mediterranean eating routine is something beyond about nourishment, however. Customary physical action and offering suppers to others are likewise significant parts.

Along with the best healthy routine, it is important to stay consistent, patient, and clear about your target.

In the process, you must avoid junk food, snacks, and even emotional eating.

## Control Emotional Eating

Fulfilling hunger is not the only reason for our easting. Very regularly, we go to nourishment when we are pushed or on edge, which can wreck your eating routine and pack on the pounds. Do you eat when you are exhausted, lonely, or worried? If yes, you are not alone. Many people around the world tend to eat when they are emotional. Sometimes we eat without even noticing the quantity of food. All these attitudes affect the target of losing weight.

The following are some of the best ways to release tension and feel fresh, active, and energetic.

**Stressed** – find more beneficial approaches to calm yourself. Attempt meditation, yoga, or absorbing a hot shower.

**Feeling down** – find other mid-evening jolts of energy. Take a stab while strolling around the square, tuning in to stimulating music, or taking a short snooze.

**Desolate or exhausted** – connect with others as opposed to going after the fridge. Make a Call to a friend who makes you snicker, go for a walk, or go to the library, shopping center, or park—anyplace there are people. Socializing is an excellent way to feel better about things.

Keep away from interruptions while eating. Also, try not to eat while working, sitting in front of the TV, or driving. It's excessively simple to overeat thoughtlessly. So, try not to distract your concentration while eating, and follow one work at a time formula. It makes things very easy and increases efficiency.

Try to eat slowly, appreciating the scents and surfaces of your nourishment. If your brain meanders, delicately return your consideration regarding your food and its taste.

Another important trick which we need to follow is we need to eat less. We must learn the art to stop eating before we are completely full. We must not be committed to clean our plates.

## Reducing the Consumption of Sugar

Regardless of whether you're explicitly planning to cut carbs, a large portion of us devours to go for sugary foods. Apart from that, refined starches and added sugar are found abundantly in many processed foods. So, it is better to avoid fast food as it contains both of them. In case you can not quit eating fast foods, it is advised to reduce the quantity or read the ingredients list posted on the pack. This will help you to have an idea of how much of added sugar or refined starches you are consuming. Vegetables and fresh fruits complete the body's needs of sugar, and these added sugars, unfortunately, convert into fats and develop spikes in your blood glucose.

Calories acquired from fructose (that are found in sugary drinks, for example, pop and canned foods like doughnuts, biscuits, and candy) are bound to add to fat around your belly. Reducing the level of sugar can mean a slimmer waistline just as a lower danger of diabetes.

Thus keeping all these things in mind, it's crucial to eat healthily rather than eat more. While we are fasting, we need to consume as per the body's need. If we eat more, it can damage health negatively. If we eat more, it is not a good sign either. So what's the solution then? We need to keep a balance between these two extremes. We need to maintain the shape as well as the energy levels of the body. It is essential to have a look at what we eat daily. Therefore, that proportion between getting obese or getting dangerously thinner is vital to maintain. We have to eat healthy food that can give us enough energy through which we can survive and have a good healthy body.

# Eat healthily and stay healthy:

Fasting has been practiced for years and is a staple across many different religions and cultures around the globe. Fasting is an act in which a person eats at the start of the day and then eats nothing the whole day until the sunset. Muslims keep fasting once in a year in the Holy month of Ramadan or on some other religious and spiritual days. They repeatedly keep fasting for the whole month. Now, the question is, how a person eats healthy but also helps in weight loss while fasting. First of all, losing weight is a difficult job for obese people. They find it hard to burn their fats. They cannot control themselves from eating three times a day. During Ramadan, they will schedule their time of eating, as they will eat early in the morning, and then for the whole day, they will not eat or drink anything. In the evening they will eat. This will prevent them from eating three times. This will help them in burning their calories the whole day.

In short, we can easily say that the benefits of fasting are life-changing. It keeps you away all day from the food. As a result, all day, you burn calories without taking any. Also, it increases the speed of your metabolism and thus you the undesired fats from your body. Lastly, it also decreases the chances of many fatal diseases, such as diabetes and sugar.

## 1: Oatmeal

Oatmeal is a nutritional powerhouse. It contains beta-glucan, which is a thick, sticky fiber that helps a person to feel energetic for more extended periods and may also lower the level of cholesterol.

Oatmeal also brings a good for those who are overweight. The studies show that those who take oatmeal in the morning felt more active and energetic. This is specifically true for people who are obese. Besides, it also helps to control the level of your blood sugar level. Therefore, it would be a nice idea to make oatmeal a regular breakfast dish.

## 2. Eggs

Eggs could be a nice little dish for you if you want to reduce your weight. It was considered that eggs contain dangerous cholesterol, but that was actually not true. The recent data tells us another story. It is concluded that basically, eggs contain good cholesterol that is good for health. Also, it is a rich source of protein, calcium. Boiled eggs are even more beneficial. It does not only give you a delicious taste, but it's incredible qualities make it a perfect choice for all those people who are seeking to reduce weight.

There is no doubt that eggs are a very popular dish for breakfast around the world, and this trend coming from an unknown period of time. Similarly, it reduces the chance of type 2 diabetes. Eggs are a popular breakfast food. They are nutritious and contain high-quality protein.

## 3. Nuts and nut butter

The benefits of nuts and its butter are incredible. It contains high-quality protein that is very heart's health. Doctors and experts have recommended that nuts actually be a suitable replacement for meat. This shows the quality and quantity of protein it contains.

Its butter could an amazing and delicious food as well. Its benefits are numerous. You can spread its butter on the bread, and that is amazing breakfast food.

Several studies have concluded that those who eat nuts regularly live longer than those who do not eat nuts. Hence, we can say that nuts can help you to stay healthy and lose weight.

Healthful kinds of nut butter include:

- Peanut butter

- Almond butter

- Cashew butter

- Unsweetened cocoa and hazelnut butter

**4. Coffee**

Coffee is widely around the world. If you stressed, tired, or exhausted, go for a cup of coffee. Not only that, but people also take coffee when they are in a good mood.

Apart from its taste, it has many health benefits as well. It improves metabolism. Also, it is immune to prevent the risk of diabetes. One must be aware that adding cream to the coffee will decrease the positive impacts of coffee on the body. Similarly, adding a lot of sugar to the coffee will also decrease the benefits of coffee. Even though coffee is not a dish, however, it can help to help your cause and weight loss.

**5. Berries**

Surely, berries can become your favorite morning food if you realized the benefits of berries. All types of berries are exceptionally useful to reduce your weight. Besides the low energy (calories) density, it is a rich source of fiber Additionally; it contains disease-fighting qualities. One survey reveals that it can reduce the risk of breast cancer in young girls.

Sprinkle berries on your cereal, oatmeal, or yogurt, or you can also blend them into smoothies. In case, the fresh berries are not available; we will recommend you to go for canned or frozen berries. One must be cautious about the added sugar in the frozen or canned berries. If you are unsure about the quantity of added sugar, it is better to read the ingredients list printed on the pack.

## 6. Flaxseed

First, flaxseed is a rich source of protein, omega-3 fatty acids, and fiber. The flaxseed can benefit you in many ways, for instance, lowering the level of cholesterol, controlling blood pressure, and even reducing the risk of breast cancer. Furthermore, it can also help you to improve the sensitivity of insulin.

It is highly advised to grind the seeds of flaxseed at home or buy ground flaxseed from the market. It is because that the seeds, without even breaking down, will pass through the body, and the body receives little nutrition out of it. On the other hand, grinned seeds gives the maximum benefit to the body.


## 7. Yogurt

Mixing bananas in yogurt could be an amazing way to start your morning with. It helps and improves the life and health of your stomach. It helps greatly to improve your digestion. If you are fasting, try yogurt in the early morning before starting the fast, at least once.

It keeps the stomach cool and gives extra energy for your day. All-day you feel good. Just like milk and other dairy product, yogurt can give a much-needed dose of protein for your body.

## 8. Tea

All type of tea is extremely beneficial; however, green tea is a time tested type of tea. It improves your blood circulation and helps you in your digestion. It is observed that green tea helps you to burn your undesired and unhealthy fats. Adding lemon to green tea is another fabulous way to burn fats and stay away from many diseases.

## 9. Cottage Cheese

It is another dish full of proteins. In case you are immune to eggs, go for cottage cheese. It could be an excellent alternate for gees. Apart from proteins, it is also a big source of calcium and vitamins.

It reduces the craving for food, which, as a result, helps you to reduce weight. Additionally, you can mix cottage cheese with other green vegetables, which makes a perfect combo of taste and health benefits.

## 10. Bananas

As we discussed in the yogurt section, the bananas are an amazing food choice for breakfast. It is a very high source of fibers and reduces the craving for foods. Adding bananas into yogurt can give you a fantastic start to your day.

Apart from that, you can replace snacks with bananas. Instead of taking snacks, go to the refrigerator and eat a banana. It not only fulfills your hunger but also is an amazingly healthy food choice.

If you have any digestion or stomach related issues, we will strongly recommend bananas as a cure for the stomach. You will surely feel the difference.

# Eat and lose weight at the same time:

### 1.   Corn

A significant number of us have extraordinary summer recollections encompassing sweet corn. In the Midwest, when sweet corn is prepared, our suppers take on an alternate look like ears of corn advance toward our plates. A few families even have a yearly occasion where a few ages get together to go through a day canning or freezing corn. In any case, there's a whole other world to corn than simply the rendition on the cob.

The corn can be classified into four categories, popcorn, sweets, and decorative, beyond what 200 assortments of corn can be discovered developing in the United States today. Corn is flexible since the whole corn plant can be utilized. You can use the husks for making tamales, the silk to make a medicinal tea, the pieces for nourishment, and the stalks for animals feed. You can discover corn in items like tortillas, tortilla chips, cornmeal, and corn oil. Smaller than usual ears of corn, known as child corn, can be utilized in hors d'oeuvres, soups, chowders, stews, and pan-fried food dishes. Infant corn is exceptionally well known in Thai and Chinese cooking.

## 2. Celery

If you are trying to lose weight, the celery is a perfect choice for you. It is highly suggested because it contains fewer calories and makes you feel full. Therefore, it is a fantastic choice for all those people who want to reduce their weight. You can eat in front of your laptop or TV screen as you will not go to sleep hungry.

## 3. Turnips

Despite the fact that it's regularly confused with an individual from the root family, the turnip originates from the cruciferous family with relations to Brussels sprouts, kale, and broccoli. It is, in any case, the bulbous foundation of the turnip that is regularly expended. As a result of this gathering, the turnip is known for its high supplement tally and its low-calorie thickness, which makes it ideal nourishment to add to your smart dieting plan. In one medium-sized turnip, there are only 34 calories, 4 grams of fiber when cooked, and 1 gram of protein. It additionally contains the greater part of your everyday nutrient. If you ever underestimated the medical benefits of turnip, we will advise you to reconsider it.

### 5.  Purple Cabbage

Purple cabbage is rich in color as well as in taste, and all of its health benefits turn it into a healthy vegetable that can be easily consumed in your evening salads. Thanks to beta-carotene, which converts itself into vitamin A when in our bodies, purple cabbage helps maintain digestive and urinary system tissue.

It also has high levels of sulfur, which allows it to contribute to cleaning the digestive system and preventing constipation. Also, it's especially recommended if you happen to be hungry at 6 PM but need to stay up late, as it helps to avoid fatigue and contributes to concentration.

## 5. Mushrooms

If you are looking for a low-calorie dish, mushrooms could be ideal for you. It is a rich source of minerals and vitamins. Besides, it also contains a significant amount of proteins. Eating of edible mushrooms decreases the craving for food and thus helps you to feel full for an extended period of time. So, if you want to reduce weight, mushrooms should be on your menu list.

## 6. Cherries

If you take soda or other beverages regularly, we will suggest you switch it with the juice of cherries. This could be an amazing healthy replacement as we all know that beverages contain a high amount of added sugar, which is never good for your health whether you are trying to reduce your weight or not. Moreover, it can help you to sleep well at night,

## 7. Beets

It is yet another excellent dish for your menu if you are trying to find dishes for the menu, which can help to lose weight. It will not only help you to reduce weight but also improve your metabolism. Likewise, it reduces hunger for more time. Therefore, it is an ideal choice for your weight-reducing food menu.

## 8. Kiwi

Kiwi is yet another amazing healthy food for your menu. It has many benefits; for example, it helps you to burn fats. It improves your digestion. It keeps the skin fresh and removes waste from your skin. As a result, your skin shines, you feel good, and your digestion is great. Lastly, it also keeps your hair healthy and shiny.

## 9. Greek Yogurt

This is a special yogurt that contrasts from different yogurts since it experiences a stressing procedure to evacuate the whey. Whey is a fluid that contains lactose, a characteristic sugar found in milk. Greek yogurt is a well-known dairy item, yet is it bravo?

Making yogurt includes aging milk with live societies of useful microorganisms.

Stressed Greek yogurt is lower in sugar than ordinary yogurt. Evacuating the whey delivers a thicker, creamier yogurt with a tart taste.

Some of the benefits of Greek yogurt are listed below.

- It improves the health of your bones

- It reduces the craving for food and snacks

- It speeds the metabolism

- Help to improve your gut health

- It impacts your mental health positively

- Helps to improve your muscles health

- Keep your blood pressure under control

- Decreases the chances of diabetes

Apart from religious rewards, fasting could be an excellent way to improve your health and reduce weight. The only condition is that one must take proper food choices while fasting.

Eat a healthy diet during your eating period and drink calorie-free beverages like water or unsweetened teas and coffee.

# Proven healthy foods for Weight-loss:

Losing weight could be problematic, time-consuming, and tiring process. It takes time and requires the sacrifice of your favorite foods. At times it becomes challenging to keep a count on the intake of calories each day. It is important to have a look at the daily consumption of calories and to burn off the calories. The reduction of weight is a time-consuming process, but patience and consistency are key. Some argue that taking fewer calories than needed is helpful to reduce weight; some say that reducing of high-fat foods can be beneficial to lose weight. Others may say that the consumption of fewer carbs is the key to reduce weight. However, with the right options, you can achieve the desired results. The most important thing is to have a look at the consumption and burning of calories.

You need to keep the intake and burning of the calories in proportion. If you are taking more calories and losing less, that is dangerous. On the other hand, if you are consuming fewer calories and burning more calories that will help you to reduce weight. Some foods are healthy but contain fewer calories. In this section, we will talk about those foods which are healthy, yet help you to reduce weight and get some amazing results. The following are the foods that are healthy and helpful to lose weight.

## 1. Whole Eggs

Once considered high in cholesterol, but recent studies show that eggs can be helpful to reduce weight. Healthy fats and protein are found abundantly in eggs. It could be an ideal dish for breakfast. Along with its delicious taste, it helps you to suppress the craving for a long time as compared to other foods. Besides, it can also help you to reduce weight.

Eggs could be a nice little dish for you if you want to reduce your weight. It was considered that eggs contain dangerous cholesterol, but that was actually not true. The recent data tells us another story. It is concluded that basically, eggs contain good cholesterol that is good for health. Also, it is a rich source of protein, calcium. Boiled eggs are even more beneficial. It does not only give you a delicious taste, but it's incredible qualities make it a perfect choice for all those people who are seeking to reduce weight.

## 2.  Boiled Potatoes

Potatoes have some amazing properties which make it a perfect dieting dish. Potatoes contain a staggeringly different scope of nutrients — a tad of nearly all that you need. There have even been records of individuals surviving on only potatoes for broadened timeframes. They are exceptionally rich from much healthy potassium. It keeps you full for more time as compared to other foods. Therefore, it is an essential food which should on the table of all those individuals who are looking for such food which can give them an ample amount of energy as well help them not to gain weight.

Boiled potatoes are among the most filling nourishments. They are exceptionally acceptable at decreasing your hunger, possibly smothering your nourishment consumption later in the day.

### 3. Soups

Those foods which have low energy density tend to make people eat fewer calories. Most nourishments with a low energy density are those that contain loads of water, for example, vegetables and other organic products. Along with that, you can also add some water to your soup. Data shows that eating the same nourishment transformed into a soup as opposed to intense nourishment, causes individuals to feel increasingly satisfied and eat fundamentally fewer calories. Simply try not to add an excessive amount of fat to your soup, for example, cream or coconut milk, as this can altogether expand its calorie content.

Soups can be a viable piece of not gaining weight diet. It has a lot of water which keeps you full for a long time. Be that as it may, attempt to stay away from creamy or smooth soups.

### 4.  Nuts

Although nuts are high in fat, nuts are not as stuffing as you would anticipate. They're a superb tidbit containing adjusted measures of protein, fiber, and solid fats. Studies have indicated that eating nuts can improve metabolic wellbeing and even advance weight reduction. Besides, the populace considers have demonstrated that individuals who eat nuts will, in general, be more advantageous and less fatty.

However, one should be cautious not to go beyond the lines as nuts are still high in calories. If you will in the wide gorge and eat large measures of nuts, it might be ideal for evading them.

Nuts can make a robust expansion to a viable weight reduction diet when devoured with some restraint.

### 5.  Whole Grains

Although oat grains have gotten awful notoriety as of late, a few sorts are unquestionably sound. The whole grains have some amount of fiber as well and contain a respectable measure of protein. Striking models incorporate oats, dark-colored rice, and quinoa. Oats are loaded with solvent filaments, beta-glucans that have been appeared to build satiety and improve metabolic health.

Both dark-colored and white rice can contain vast measures of safe starch, especially whenever cooked and afterward permitted to cool a while later.

Remember that refined grains are not a sound decision, and now and then nourishments that have "entire grains" on the name are profoundly prepared low-quality nourishments that are both not helpful and stuff. In case you're on a low-carb diet, you'll need to keep away from grains, as they're high in carbs. However, there's, in any case, nothing amiss with eating entire grains in the event that you can endure them.

You ought to stay away from refined grains in case you're attempting to lose weight. Pick entire grains instead — they're a lot higher in fiber and different supplements.

## 6. Fruits

Almost all health experts agree that fruits are healthy. Various researches have indicated that individuals who eat the most products of the soil will, in general, be more beneficial than individuals who don't.

Obviously, the relationship doesn't rise to causation, so these examinations don't demonstrate anything. Notwithstanding, natural products do possess properties that make them weight reduction amicable. Despite the fact that they contain sugar, they have a low energy density and require a significant period to bite. Besides, their fiber content keeps sugar from being discharged too rapidly into your circulation system. The individuals who might need to stay away from or limit organic products are those on an extremely low-carb, ketogenic count calories or have a prejudice.

We can say that fruits are delicious and could be useful in weight reduction.

In spite of the fact that organic products contain some sugar, you can, without much of a stretch, remember them for a weight reduction diet. It provides a high amount of fiber. Lastly, it can also prevent several types of cancer.

### 7.  Coconut Oil

All the fats are not the same. Experts have agreed to classify fats into two categories. The first one is good fats (unsaturated fats), while the other one is bad fats or saturated fats. The coconut is a rich source of good fats or unsaturated fats. These good fats have been appeared to help satiety better than different fats and increment the number of calories consumed. In addition, two investigations — one in ladies and the other in men — indicated that coconut oil decreased measures of tummy fat. Obviously, coconut oil, despite everything, contains calories. Therefore, coconut oil should be limited, as it can affect you adversely.

Finally, it is worth mentioning that virgin olive oil is perhaps the most beneficial fat on earth.


### 8.  Yogurt

Yogurt is phenomenal dairy nourishment. Specific sorts of yogurt contain probiotic microorganisms that can improve the capacity of your gut. Having a solid gut may help secure against irritation and leptin obstruction, which is one of the basic reasons for weight gain. Furthermore, make a note to get yogurt with live, as different sorts of yogurt contain no probiotics.

Similarly, think of picking creamy yogurt. Data shows that creamy yogurt — however, not low-fat — is related to a decreased danger of obesity and type 2 diabetes after some time. Low-fat yogurt is usually stacked with sugar, so it's ideal for keeping away from it. Probiotic yogurt can impact your digestive system positively. Consider adding it to your weight reduction diet yet make a point to maintain a strategic distance from items that contain included sugar.

Protein usually is filling and takes more time to process than basic sugars. When people opt for a whey protein drink, they shed around 4 pounds more and about an inch more from their midsections more than a half year and felt less eager than individuals given a starch shake. Other research in mice, found that when mice were given extra whey protein, they got less weight and muscle to the ratio obesity and increasingly slender muscle, in any event, when calories were the equivalent. Whey protein is found generally in yogurt and other dairies.

Spare calories and superfluous sugar by picking plain yogurt. You can add some fresh fruits for sweetness. However, one must be cautious about the packaged yogurt as it may contain added sugar and high-fats. Try to read the ingredients label before eating.

### 9. Beans & Legumes

It is said that if you can not eat meat due to some reason, the beans could be a fitting replacement. It gives almost the same amount of energy as meat provides. There are various types of beans, and all of them are a very significant source of protein. Just like other dishes that we discussed, the beans have the same quality to reduce hunger and keep you craving away for the late day. It gives a feeling of satisfaction as far as hunger is concerned.

Apart from proteins, it is also loaded with fiber and some amount of safe starch. It is a nice option for your weight-reducing diet as it gives an ample amount of energy. With the help of that energy, you would feel strong and energetic all day. Finally, you would feel full while consuming fewer calories.

## 10. Lean Beef and Chicken Breast

Meat has been unreasonably derided. Beef is accused of many health issues regardless of the absence of proper proof to back up these negative cases. In spite of the fact that processed meat is unhealthy, studies show that natural red meat doesn't raise the danger of coronary diseases or diabetes. As indicated by two major studies, red meat has more negative health effects on men than women.

Meat is a weight reduction benevolent nourishment since it is loaded with protein.

Protein helps your hunger for a long time. Therefore, it can facilitate you to take almost 100 fewer calories daily. It also removes the craving for hunger, which saves you from regular snacking and chocolate eating.

If you intend to take low carbohydrates, lean meat is a perfect choice. It gives you energy for the whole day. Taking meat in your diet will increase the amount of protein, which makes it easier to lose weight.

### 11. Bananas

Bananas are a phenomenal wellspring of fiber. A medium banana contains 3.07 grams (g) of fiber, and the suggested day by day consumption for grown-ups is 25 g for those on a 2,000-calorie diet.

Research shows that there is a connection between higher fiber consumption and lower body loads. This supplement may likewise help decrease and settle glucose levels. Fiber can assist individuals with feeling full for more time, which may lessen the number of calories that they eat. The body sets aside an extended effort to process specific sorts of fiber, permitting it to direct nourishment consumption better. The creators of a survey that took a gander at more than 50 investigations propose that expanding the everyday intake of fiber by 14 g could prompt a 10% reduction in by and large vitality consumption and a weight reduction of 2 kilograms (4.41 pounds) more than four months.

Researches from China took a gander at the impacts of dietary fiber on craving in 100 overweight yet, in any case, sound grown-ups. The outcomes demonstrated that an expansion in dietary fiber diminished sentiments of craving, just as what number of calories the members devoured. Fiber may likewise help lower cholesterol levels and lessen the danger of coronary diseases.

Unripe green bananas contain safe starch. Safe starch is a sugar that doesn't separate effectively in the small digestive tract. Rather, it goes through to the large intestine, which implies that it doesn't expand glucose levels. It, at that point, ages in the digestive organ, animating the development of good microbes in the gut. Eating increasingly safe starch may assist individuals with getting in shape, as it acts along these lines to dietary fiber. It might diminish an individual's hunger by making them feel more full for more time. The research proposes that safe starch could likewise help improve insulin affectability. The advantages that it accommodates gut wellbeing can help with clogging and decrease the danger of colon malignancy.

After discussing all the best healthy diets, we can say that the key to getting maximum results is patience and consistency. We need to follow a strict diet and calculate the intake and burning of the calories. Similarly, we also need to avoid high-fats, which can potentially impact your efforts in losing weight. In the same manner, the reduction of carbs in daily intake is another crucial factor to help us to lose weight.

Keeping in mind all these dietary patterns, the value of exercise can be underestimated. Exercise helps us to burn calories in our intake. Therefore, it is vital to focus on daily exercise. Experts recommend at least 30 minutes of daily exercise. That will surely help you to burn your fats & calories, and as a result, we will feel more fit and slim. Apart from physical benefits, exercise can also help you to get rid off stress and anxiety. Besides, regular exercise means better sleep at night.

# 10 Best Weight Reduction Tips

To begin with, if you get some diet book and it will pretend that it has all the answers to succeed and lose the weight you want. Some argue that the key is to eat less and exercise more; others think that low-fat is the only way to go, while others describe cutting carbohydrates. So what do you think?

The reality is that there is no "one-size-fits-all" solution for permanent healthy weight loss. What works for a person might not be exactly the same for you, as our bodies respond differently to different varieties of foods, depending on genetics and other health indicators. To find the right weight-loss method for you, it may take some time and require patience, dedication, and some experience of different foods and diets.

While some people respond well to calorie calculation or similar restrictive procedures, others respond better to having more freedom when planning weight loss plans and ideas. The freedom to avoid fried foods or reduce refined carbohydrates can lead to their success. So do not feel particularly frustrated if a diet that works for someone else is not working for you. And don't beat yourself if it is proven that the food is too restrictive for you. In the end, the diet is only for you if it is one that you can stick to overtime.

Remember: While there is no simple solution to losing weight, there are many steps you can take yourself for developing a healthy relationship with food, reduce emotional triggers for overeating, and achieve a healthy weight.

Obesity leads to so many medical issues such as diabetes, high blood pressure, stroke, heart disease, and not to mention the physical disability. Our pride is in pain in the joints that people eventually end up developing earlier in their life. People who are obese and overweight now losing weight will help you feel better to look better and get you the compliments that you want.  Obesity is preventable in the first place and also credible, and if you follow these simple, practical, and doable steps coming up next, you can have amazing results.

So, the question is how to lose weight? Here I won't be telling you to do something extreme like a thousand sit-ups a day. However, if we mix the exercise with the tips we are going to discuss, it will yield some fantastic results. There are many approaches to reduce weight while and remain healthy. Some argue that taking fewer calories than needed is the best way to the reduction of weight. Some argue otherwise, according to them, not taking fats is a workable and practical idea to lose weight. Others stress the importance of exercise for getting the best results for losing weight. They all have some genuine arguments to support their claims. Let's discuss some useful tips for losing weight.

I want you to promise yourself today that you will apply these methods, and I promise you will see incredible results. You will be losing 10, 20, 30, 40, or even a hundred pounds and you will keep it up you will love the way you are eating you will enjoy the new lifestyle, and you will keep this weight off as well.

## Tip No 1

First and foremost, the recommendation of the doctors is that if you want to reduce weight, reduce the daily intake of calories. If you cut the daily number of calories by 500, you will get astonishing results. Approximately you will lose two kilograms of weight every two months.

To achieve this target, one must be consistent and patient. You need to calculate and monitor the intake of calories closely. For this, in the first place, you have to avoid snacks. It means that you will eat only three meals a day and no snacks in between.

If you are eating snacks in between the meals, most likely, you will this target. It is so because the snacks give extra calories, and if you are not up to the task, it could fire back. Instead of losing weight, that could convert into fats.

Similarly, if you followed this trick, the mentioned number of weight reduction is guaranteed.
Therefore, it is vital not to eat anything between the meals, and wait for the next meal to arrive at the designated time. It will not only help to increase your hunger but also, it will develop routine and fixed timings for the meal.

**Tip No 2**

It is about portion size, so you don't need to change what you eat, but you are going to have to change your portion size. You have to reduce the consumption of food on a daily basis. In other words, you must not be committed to clean the plate.

It is observed that when someone is served with the food on the table, they eat more. On the other hand, if someone is served with less, in most cases, they do not ask for a second refilling.

You can also follow this strategy of serving less. It is all about habit development. Once you get used to it, you will be comfortable with it.

**Tip No 3**

The third tip is to avoid snacks between the meals. Try to eat on the specific but not between the meals. Try to promise yourself that in any case, you will never eat anything between the meals.

It is extremely easy to follow, as you need just slight adjustments. You have to be committed that you do not have to eat snacks, biscuits, and especially fast-foods. Fast food consists of high-fats and added sugar. Therefore, there is no room for snacks and fast food.

All the groups showed great results, but the clear winner of this study was the first group, the diet control group, so after six weeks, there was a discount of 5 centimeters in the waistline. There were also improvements in certain health parameters like blood pressure, blood glucose, and lipids. After all this study, if you were to mix the abdominal workout group with the diet control group, then just imagine the results.

It is a doable job to reduce weight just by taking fewer calories and avoid sugary and high-fat foods. However, if you add exercise to your diet plan, that would be a win-win situation. You will surely get the desired results, and the reduction of weight will be visible within a few weeks.

**Tip No 4**

You are not going to drink juice, especially juice that you buy at the grocery store. That packaged juice is bad for you as in every situation because it is filled with added sugar, and you need to avoid sugar. Now, we are going to discuss in terms of teaspoons of sugar so you can relate to it. One glass of orange juice contains five teaspoons of sugar. It is always better to eat the fruit instead of drinking juice, especially if it is packaged. If it comes in a carton or if it is bottled, so it is better to avoid juices. Packaged and canned juices contain added sugar, and this is exactly what we need to avoid. We must opt for fresh fruits and juices. Along with its delicious taste, it gives us enough calories to work with.

**Tip No 5**

You have to avoid soda and carbonated drinks. I know that it is not an easy job, but it is not that difficult either. In a regular 12 ounce can of soda, there could be eight teaspoons of sugar. Probably, you would think that you consume zero-calorie drinks, and you think you can drink all you want, but keep in mind these usually have artificial sweeteners, which work to fool your body and fool your pancreas. Likewise, as we mentioned in the previous tip, the carbonated drinks come with added sugar. We need o to consume as little sugar as possible. Hence, it is important not to consume soda and carbonated drinks.

I believe that you should always be honest with yourself, whether it is your health, your emotions, or your abilities, and likewise. Therefore, don't fool your body nor your hormonal system; nothing good can ever come out of it.

**Tip No 6**

Try to eat your dinner at 6 p.m., and no food goes into your mouth after 6:30 p.m. You need the food to be initially used up by some activity before your sleep, so give yourself ample time. If you eat too close to bedtime, all the calories will end up being stored as fat, which is exactly what you don't need. Physical activity is crucial after dinner. There are two solutions. First, try to eat in the evening, so it gives your stomach enough time before sleeping to digest the food. Secondly, if it is difficult for you to eat your dinner so early in the evening, then make sure not to sleep right after dinner. You can go for a walk to a nearby park, or visit the market near you. It will prevent all the calories from converting to fats, and you can not afford to convert calories into fats. Instead, you need to do exactly the opposite, burn the fats.

**Tip No 7**

Do this right now, throw away your regular meal plates and go out and get smaller plates. Eat as much as you want in those plates, but don't go for a second refilling. If you eat in big bowls, go and buy smaller pots at the earliest. After doing all this stuff, you will be starving for your next meal, and you will enjoy the food you eat.

It has been observed that sometimes we eat to size of the pot. It is all about practice and routine. If you get used to the smaller plate, believe me after some time you will be comfortable to go with that smaller pots. Therefore, it is critical to replace the bigger bowls and plates with the smaller ones as it will you not to overeat. Although it seems a little awkward, the results will be astonishing, all you need just to keep patience and consistency.

**Tip No 8**

This is an indisputable fact that regular exercise can play a vital role in losing weight, improving health results, and decreasing dangers of interminable conditions, for example, diabetes and coronary illness. Correspondingly to nourishment decisions, it's significant that you try and discover the activity you appreciate! Regardless of whether it's lifting loads, interim preparing, or oxygen-consuming activities like running, biking, moving, and other cardio exercises, any physical movement that makes you move is worth your time. Try not to stress yourself out over finding the ideal exercise plan, and don't succumb to the fantasy that the "right" physical action will soften away gut fat. Simply get going, and you'll begin seeing the advantages of exercise.

You might be wondering, how might I get more fit quick without work out? Even though exercise can assist, it is conceivable with losing weight without exercise. Keep in mind, melting fats is about caloric equalization. Exercise helps in weight reduction since exercise consumes calories. To shed weight without exercise, it's critical to know about the measure of calories you are eating every day.

Exercise isn't just about oxygen consuming limit and muscle size. Of course, exercise can improve your physical wellbeing and your body, trim your waistline, improve your sexual coexistence, and even add a long time to your life. In any case, that is not what rouses the vast majority to remain active. Individuals who practice routinely will, in general, do so on the grounds that it gives them a tremendous feeling of prosperity. They feel progressively energetic for the duration of the day, rest better at night time, have more keen recollections, and feel increasingly satisfied and positive about themselves and their lives. What's more, it's likewise incredible medication for some, regular psychological health difficulties.

Therefore, the importance of exercise is irreplaceable as it helps you to burn fats. You look better and feel better. This helps you to sleep well in the night and wake up fresh in the morning. Thus, exercise keeps you active, fresh, and energetic all day.

## Tip No 9

Other than being delightful, leafy foods can assume a crucial job in weight reduction. There are nothing of the sort as otherworldly weight reduction nourishments. The significance of vegetables in weight reduction is basically founded on caloric consumption.

Fruits and vegetables incorporate fiber and a lot of water, which can assist you with feeling full while as yet devouring fewer calories. Matching leafy foods up with fit proteins and moderate sound fats can be an ideal equalization that encourages you to remain full and recuperate from your exercise. Try your level best to avoid refined carbohydrates, pasta, bread, rice, cereal cakes, and candy, the more you reduce, the quicker you will lose weight. Additionally, put more vegetables and salads on your plate, start eating cucumbers, carrots, broccoli instead of bread or rice. Eating vegetables not only helps you lose weight but also could be the perfect replacement for other high-fat recipes. Therefore, the value of vegetables is significant. Apart from that, you also need to drink at least eight glasses of water daily.

**Tip No. 10**

The final but most crucial step is fasting. Despite the recent surge in its popularity, its origin can be traced in ancient times. It has been practiced for many centuries throughout different ages, cultures, and religions. Fasting is one of the most effective ways to lose weight. If you do not eat anything from dawn to dusk, so how can you gain weight. People around the world keep fasting one way another but mostly for religious reasons. We will not go into the details of its spiritual purifications; however, it is clear that along with countless medical and physical benefits, it brings mental clarity. Ancient Greeks used to fast for this specific reason.

There is some acceptable, logical proof recommending that circadian cadence fasting, when joined with a sound eating regimen and way of life, can be an especially powerful way to deal with weight reduction, particularly for individuals in danger for diabetes. (In any case, individuals with cutting edge diabetes or who are on meds for diabetes, individuals with a background marked by dietary problems like anorexia and bulimia, and pregnant or breastfeeding ladies ought not to endeavor irregular fasting except if under the nearby supervision of a doctor who can screen them.)

Fasting is just like skipping your lunch and taking dinner in the evening. This is a beautiful routine as far as health is concerned. It gives enough time to your tummy to digest the food eaten in the evening. A heavy and healthy breakfast in the morning, and then not eating until the sunset can help you to burn your fats significantly. Although it is a religious practice, many scientific pieces of research have proved that fasting has numerous medical and health benefits. The loss of weight is on the top of the tree.

# Conclusion

Eating healthy food is not rocket science. On the off chance, when you feel overwhelmed by all the clashing advice and diet counsel out there, you are not the only one. It appears that for each expert who reveals to you specific nourishment is beneficial for you, you will discover another maxim precisely the inverse. In all actuality, while some particular nourishments or supplements have been appeared to affect temperament beneficially, it's your general dietary example that is generally significant. The foundation of a solid eating routine ought to be to supplant processed food with natural fresh food at whatever point conceivable. Eating nourishment that is as close as credible to nature can make a big difference in how you think, look, and feel. Try to keep your goals modest, and aim for one target at a time. This strategy will surely help you in the long run, if followed accurately.

www.ingramcontent.com/pod-product-compliance
Lightning Source LLC
Chambersburg PA
CBHW031111250726
48655CB00004B/1661